YOUR BREASTFEEDING COACH

The Help You Need for Successful Breastfeeding

Jill Lindquist

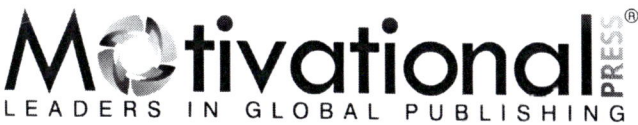

Published by Motivational Press, Inc.
7777 N Wickham Rd, # 12-247
Melbourne, FL 32940
www.MotivationalPress.com

Copyright © by Jill Lindquist

All Rights Reserved

No part of this book may be reproduced or transmitted in any form by any means: graphic, electronic, or mechanical, including photocopying, recording, taping or by any information storage or retrieval system without permission, in writing, from the authors, except for the inclusion of brief quotations in a review, article, book, or academic paper. The authors and publisher of this book and the associated materials have used their best efforts in preparing this material. The authors and publisher make no representations or warranties with respect to accuracy, applicability, fitness or completeness of the contents of this material. They disclaim any warranties expressed or implied, merchantability, or fitness for any particular purpose. The authors and publisher shall in no event be held liable for any loss or other damages, including but not limited to special, incidental, consequential, or other damages. If you have any questions or concerns, the advice of a competent professional should be sought.

Manufactured in the United States of America.

ISBN:

Contents

Dedications 5
Introduction 7

Series Book #1: Giving Your Baby the Best; Your Breast Milk
Chapter 1: Why should I breastfeed? 9
Chapter 2: What does breast milk have that's so special for my baby? 11
Chapter 3: What's so special about breastfeeding for me? 14
Chapter 4: Can I produce enough milk for my baby? 16
Chapter 5: Can I still breastfeed if I've had breast surgery? 19
Chapter 6: Can I still breastfeed if my baby takes a bottle? 21
Chapter 7: How do medications and alcohol affect the breast milk? 23

Series Book #2: Helpful Hints Before You Deliver
Chapter 8: What's a Midwife, Doula or Lactation Consultant? 26
Chapter 9: What should I look for when choosing a hospital? 29
Chapter 10: What is donor milk and is it safe? 31
Chapter 11: What should I look for when choosing a breast pump? 33
Chapter 12: Is Daddy feeling left out? 35
Chapter 13: Is your support system in place? 38
Chapter 14: What type of birth control is best when I'm breastfeeding? ..41

Series Book #3: Baby's Here! The First Days
Chapter 15: How do I get off to a great start? 44
Chapter 16: What are the best positions for successful breastfeeding? 47
Chapter 17: How do I know if I have a good latch? 50
Chapter 18: I had a rough delivery; what can I expect now? 54
Chapter 19: How much nipple pain is normal? 59
Chapter 20: How do I know I have enough milk for my baby? 63
Chapter 21: What if my baby needs to be supplemented? 66

Book Series #4: What Should I Do Now? Your Troubleshooting Guide
Chapter 22: What should I do when my breasts are engorged? 69
Chapter 23: What should I do if my baby isn't gaining weight? ... 72
Chapter 24: What should I do if I have too much milk? 78
Chapter 25: I think I have plugged ducts or mastitis or thrush.
   What should I do? 83

    Chapter 26: Would using a nipple shield help my situation? 88
    Chapter 27: I have so many more questions, where should I start? 91

Book Series #5: Low Milk Supply ~ Actual Answers with Real Results
    Chapter 28: How do I know if I have a low milk supply? 96
    Chapter 29: What are some reasons I might not produce enough milk? ..99
    Chapter 30: Can I correct my problem and increase
                   my low milk supply? 104
    Chapter 31: What foods can I eat that would help increase
                   my milk supply? 106
    Chapter 32: What herbals might help increase my milk supply? 110
    Chapter 33: What choices are there other than combination herbals? 113

Book Series #6: When Unexpected Situations Separate You and Baby
    Chapter 34: I wasn't expecting this, what happens now? 118
    Chapter 35: My baby is early and so very small, how can I help them? ...121
    Chapter 36: What can I expect when my baby starts to breastfeed? 125
    Chapter 37: I have so many different emotions,
                   how can I process them? 129
    Chapter 38: We're going home! Will I know what to do? 133

Book Series #7: Back to work ~ You Can Do It!
    Chapter 39: What rights do I have when I return to work? 136
    Chapter 40: What are the benefits to my baby and me
                   when I provide pumped milk? 138
    Chapter 41: What are the benefits to my employer
                   when I pump at work? 140
    Chapter 42: What do I need to be prepared for pumping at work? 142
    Chapter 43: What is the best way to store pumped milk? 147

Bibliography 149
Articles 149
Websites 150
Videos 151

About the Author 154

Dedications

I dedicate this book to Evelyn Lindholm and Ardys Christenson.

Evelyn, you are one of the most sincere and kindhearted persons I have ever had the privilege of knowing. Our time together as business partners, co-workers and friends has been a great joy in my life. You have helped me grow in ways I never knew possible and encouraged me to become someone I never knew I could be. I am forever grateful to you for your friendship and the gifts you bring to mothers and babies.

Ardys, your assistance with this project has been an enormous help of which I am most thankful for. The hours you spent pouring over the content and providing feedback was invaluable. Your dedication to this book and the belief this will help breastfeeding mothers everywhere has touched my heart. Your passion for babies and your compassion for mothers is a gift you continue to share. I am eternally grateful for you and your talents.

Introduction

The decision to breastfeed your baby is a big one, no doubt. There are different opinions and plenty of advice from well-meaning people. You may also find confusion and mixed messages as you research this decision. How do you keep it all straight and sift through the information to find what's best for you? I am a Lactation Consultant and a Registered Nurse with nearly 20 years of experience in the field of lactation. I've worked in several different metro area hospitals assisting mothers with all aspects of breastfeeding. I've also worked with mothers in a variety of settings; from hospitals, home births, home care, and follow up phone calls to outpatient support and consultation. I'm here to help you sort it all out; why breastfeeding is truly best-feeding. I have written this book as a helper or 'coach' for you, the mother. I cover topics such as, why breastfeeding is so important for you and your baby, why skin to skin can make a big impact on your success and overall experience, trouble-shooting through difficult moments including low milk supply and returning to work successfully. I have also made the topics in this book available as an eBook SERIES. Perhaps you may have a need for only 3 or 4 topics. You can find these topics available under 'Your Breastfeeding Coach'. My wish is you will find this book helpful as you navigate your way through your breastfeeding experience. It was written for you the mother, to help you along your journey. Take the time to enjoy this moment in your life. The moment of being a mom, nursing your baby and creating a relationship like none you've ever known. It's an experience you will never forget. Congratulations and best of luck to you.

Jill

Chapter 1: Why should I breastfeed?

Deciding to breastfeed is one of the biggest decisions you will face now that you are expecting a baby. I found when researching articles, books and pamphlets about breastfeeding that there wasn't much out there that was easy to get your hands on to help you make this decision. I hope this will help clear things up for you and show you that not only is your breast milk the best food for your baby, breastfeeding is also very doable with a little support and education.

Your baby gets wonderful immunity they can't get anywhere else when breastfeeding. Throughout the duration of your life your body has been building up antibodies against colds, flus and other diseases. An antibody is a part of your immune system, which helps identify and fight bacteria and viruses. All these wonderful antibodies from your body are present in your breast milk, giving your baby protection from disease every time they nurse.

Your breast milk provides precisely what your baby needs, exactly when they need it. Your breast milk is species specific and made just for them and their needs. Your baby will regulate how much milk they need by how often they eat and their nursing style. Your body receives all the messages it needs to provide milk for your baby. Mother Nature is very strong! Breast milk is living fluid you make continuously and individually for each baby.

Do you want to save hundreds of dollars each month? Yes, breastfeeding is economical as well. When researching the amount of money it costs to provide formula to your baby, the answers varied slightly. Because not every baby consumes the same amount of ounces of formula per year, I have taken a yearly average. Based on the average, cost of formula per month is $300. That becomes $3,600.00 per year you can save by breastfeeding your baby.

What an amazing process! Your baby gets immunities from you that they can never receive from anything else, even donor milk. You provide exactly what your baby needs, when they need it, all while saving thousands of dollars. The benefits don't stop there. Starting your baby off with a healthy digestive system plays an important role for their future health. We will explore more in the next chapter.

Chapter 2: What does breast milk have that's so special for my baby?

Your breast milk contains so much more than you could ever imagine. Sometimes it can be hard to believe that your body can do all this without you even knowing it. Your baby will continue to receive these benefits as long as you keep providing breast milk. So breastfeed away, knowing your body is hard at work and your baby is getting all the benefits. There are so many good elements and advantages in your breast milk. You are actually preparing your baby for life-long health.

Did you know that breastfeeding helps improve your baby's cognitive development in their brain? Cognitive development is the ability to think and understand. This helps your baby in all aspects of their life. Cognitive development covers many aspects of human growth, including reasoning, vision and language recognition just to name a few.

Stem cells are the "gems" of breast milk. These cells are undifferentiated; meaning they have not become a specialized cell, or have not found a home yet. These cells are not yet "liver" cells or "muscle" cells. Researchers have discovered three different types of stem cells in breast milk, which is very unique. When your baby receives your breast milk, their little body will "direct traffic" and tell each stem cell where it will help their body the most. This is so important to a new little baby who is making the transition to life outside of their mother.

The first milk your baby receives, also called colostrum, is loaded with 50,000 stem cells per milliliter; a milliliter is about 1/5th of a teaspoon. This is exactly what your baby needs to help make this transition to independent life. Stem cells continue to be present in your mature milk. There are still 100 stem cells per milliliter of mature milk. This process continues as long as your baby receives your breast milk.

Another benefit of breast milk is that it helps protect your baby's intestinal system the moment it hits their stomach. Breast milk lines your baby's gut with a protective coating preventing diarrhea and abdominal cramping. Colostrum coats the gut right after birth with their first feeding, no waiting!

All babies are born with an immature digestive system. Their gut or digestive system is permeable, allowing liquids and gases to pass through, leaving your baby at risk of developing diarrhea and allergies. Your breast milk coats their gut, protecting and maturing it, keeping the gut more acidic which reduces the bacteria. When a baby receives even one formula feeding, this changes the entire balance of the gut. It will take at least 2-4 weeks to return the gut to its desirable state. This is an even bigger challenge with premature and sick babies, and is the number one reason neonatologists prefer breast milk for these fragile digestive systems.

Breast milk also helps prevent childhood obesity. There are 5 specific "anti-obesity" hormones present in your breast milk. Not only is your baby receiving these hormones, but your child will also learn proper eating habits right from birth. They eat when they are hungry and stop when they are full. The baby makes the decision when they are done, not the person who is giving them a bottle. The ideas of "finish the whole bottle" or "clean your plate" are often the route to later problems with managing obesity. The baby deciding when they are done is always the best measure of a healthy appetite.

Breastfeeding has also shown to lower the risk of SIDS: Sudden Infant Death Syndrome. It decreases the risk of ear infections, colds and flu; as well as the risk of childhood leukemia and childhood onset diabetes. It has been shown to increase intelligence. That is just a sample of all the benefits your breast milk provides to your baby.

Isn't it amazing what your body can do? These benefits last a lifetime; benefits that you, and you alone, can give to your baby. The satisfaction you will have is like no other you have experienced. It's important to see that even some breastfeeding or breast milk is crucial to the development of your child. Laying this groundwork early on will set your child up for the healthiest beginning possible. I'm fairly certain that scientists will discover even more perks of breast milk in the near future. I haven't forgotten about you! The benefits don't end with your baby; you get an abundance of benefits as well!

Chapter 3: What's so special about breastfeeding for me?

That's a great question! Exactly what is so special about breastfeeding for you, the mother? As a new parent or a repeat parent, you will notice much of the focus is on the baby. But we can't forget who is doing all the work. This entire chapter is devoted to the benefits for you. We wouldn't want you to get lost in the shuffle!

When you breastfeed, your uterus returns to its pre-pregnant state more quickly and you experience less blood loss. The two main hormones involved in breastfeeding are oxytocin, which contracts the milk ducts and prolactin, which makes the milk. When your baby nurses oxytocin tightens the milk ducts and releases the milk to your baby. In addition, oxytocin contracts your uterus, helping to shrink it down to its pre-pregnant state, which is about the size of your fist. This results in a flatter tummy quicker! By contracting your uterus so efficiently, this also helps prevent heavy bleeding or even hemorrhaging after delivery.

Breastfeeding can also help protect you against breast and ovarian cancer. The longer you nurse, the more protection you will receive. Estrogen is a hormone that fuels 80% of all breast cancers. When you are breastfeeding, your estrogen levels are reduced therefore decreasing your risk of breast cancer. Some research also states that while your breasts are lactating, your breast cells change and are more resistant to cancer-related mutations. You also receive protection against ovarian cancer. Most women do not ovulate while breastfeeding and experts agree that women who ovulate less often have a decreased risk of ovarian cancer. Most research shows a decreased risk by one third if you breastfeed for a total of

18 months collectively between all your breastfeeding experiences. This sounds like a win-win situation!

Osteoporosis is a medical condition where bones become brittle and fragile. Many people feel they are at risk for this when they breastfeed as the baby "takes the calcium" away from mom. This is a myth. Actually, non-breastfeeding women have a four times greater chance of developing osteoporosis than breastfeeding mothers. According to the NIH Osteoporosis and Related Bone Diseases National Resource Center, breastfeeding mothers often have stronger bones than those who have never breastfed.

Would you like to lose your extra baby weight without extra exercise? Sounds like a trick question doesn't it? I'm here to tell you this is no joke. Your body burns 300-500 calories, or more, per day making breast milk for your baby. La Leche League Breastfeeding Answer Book states that breastfeeding mothers lose more weight than bottle-feeding mothers, even if the bottle feeding mothers consume fewer calories. They go on to say that with exclusive breastfeeding, mothers have an average decrease in body fat and in hip and lower thigh circumference. You can't beat that!

There is much more to breastfeeding than I've mentioned. The psychological, social and emotional aspects you both receive cannot be measured. Breastfeeding provides a unique interaction between you and your baby. The skin-to-skin nurturing and closeness cannot be replicated. Breastfeeding provides you with regular time for resting and relaxing with your baby, as the two of you grow close, develop a relationship with each other and begin an emotional bond that lasts a lifetime. Like I said, you can't beat those benefits!

Sometimes I wish I were breastfeeding again. It was a very magical time for my children and I one I will never forget! Knowing your body is protecting you against some long-term illnesses is pretty amazing. Putting some odds in your favor can't hurt. Some of you will question your body's abilities and even wonder if you will be able to make enough milk to meet your baby's needs. The next chapter will give you all the answers and squash all those myths.

Chapter 4: Can I produce enough milk for my baby?

Most women will question their ability to produce enough milk for their baby at some point during their breastfeeding experience. For many moms this doubt begins right away, within hours after delivery. Ladies, here is the truth; there is a very slim percent of women who cannot produce enough milk for their baby. Lactation consultants have helped millions of women and I am here to assure you that you will make enough milk. With coaching, guidance and what you learn as you read, you can see your dreams and goals of breastfeeding your baby become a reality.

Inside your breasts are special nerves called receptors that sense prolactin, the primary hormone that makes milk and is regulated by the pituitary gland. These nerves will set the stage for producing enough milk. The more nerves that can be activated the better. A majority of this activation occurs in the first few days after birth. This is why it's so important in the early days of breastfeeding to allow your baby to nurse 8-10 times per day, or as often as they desire. This pattern is designed to help you with your long-term supply.

Sending your baby to the nursery for the nights after you deliver is a critical "mistaken idea" which sets you up for producing less milk. You'll see from the story below how the better choice for this mother would have been to have the baby brought to her on demand, when he was hungry or to keep him in the room with her so he can be fed easily while mom and baby get to know one another.

A mother called me frantically after her first night home from the hospital. She thought something was wrong with her baby because he "ate every two hours". When asked what her nighttime feedings were like while she was in the hospital for four days after her cesarean birth, she simply stated, "I don't know. I slept for 8 hours every night. The nurses said I should get my sleep while I could." Needless to say no good came from this advice. Not only did the mother have a delay in milk production due to a lack of stimulation and receptor growth, she also wasn't familiar with her babies' normal pattern of nighttime feedings. She was amazed at his feeding frequency and her lack of production. An aggressive feeding and stimulation plan began with this mother. She began to frequently nurse her baby, pump after nursing to help make up for the deficit, and supplement her breastfeeding. This feeding plan lasted for five days before her supply caught up with the baby's demand. So you can see how much more work was necessary because of this poor advice.

Remember your baby will tell your body how much milk to make. Getting to know these feeding patterns early and following the baby's feeding cues will start you on the road to successful breastfeeding and breast milk supply right away. The basic principle is simple: the more your baby nurses, the more your body will produce.

Along with the receptors, prolactin, the milk-making hormone, is also important to your supply success. The amount of prolactin in your body increases during pregnancy to about 10-20 times your non-pregnant levels. After the baby is born prolactin levels remain elevated for a period of time. If no stimulation occurs, the levels drop. Here are some basic levels to help give you an idea just how important early stimulation is to your milk supply:

- Non-pregnant: 10-20 ng/ml
- Immediately after birth: 300-400 ng/ml
- Seven days after birth: 100-200 ng/ml
- One month after birth: 100 ng/ml

Seeing how quickly these levels drop demonstrates the importance of breastfeeding and establishing your milk supply right after delivery.

You can see how important it is to capitalize on those very crucial days right after delivery. The mother mentioned previously would have likely avoided the entire feeding plan including pumping, supplementing, bottle washing and worrying if she would have nursed her baby on demand; day and night.

Getting off on the right foot, knowing what to expect and being an advocate for yourself and your baby can make all the difference. It's important to know the breastfeeding experience begins right away. A delay in breastfeeding could result in "jumping through more hoops" later.

Some of you might be wondering if you can breastfeed. Perhaps you didn't have success with a previous breastfeeding experience or have had some type of breast surgery. I will discuss these situations in this next chapter.

Chapter 5: Can I still breastfeed if I've had breast surgery?

Some types of breast surgeries are quite compatible with successful breastfeeding. Here are some important aspects to consider.

What if you've had breast implants? How will this affect your milk supply? Usually having breast implants doesn't affect milk supply. Surgeons typically go beneath the pectus muscle through an incision under the breast or along side the breast near the armpit for implants. This leaves all the milk ducts and sinuses intact for successful breastfeeding. The success of breastfeeding may be connected to the reason why you had the enhancement. Women have said, "I had no breasts at all," or "I looked like a 12 year old boy." There may be a chance you did not have enough glandular tissue to begin with. These mothers will likely produce milk, but may have issues with a full supply. If you had average size breasts but just wanted an enhancement, you will likely be fine.

What if you've had breast reduction surgery? How will this affect your supply? Breast reduction surgery removes tissue and skin from the breast to reduce and reshape the size of the breast. There are generally two types of procedures for breast reduction surgery. It will depend on which type of surgery you had that will likely determine the impact on breast milk production.

The first procedure most commonly used is called the Pedicle Method. This method, sometimes called the anchor method, helps to reduce breast tissue volume, contours the breast and maintains nipple function and sensation. This procedure involves raising the nipple and areola to higher positions while leaving portions of underlying tissue attached for support. The more tissue that remains intact, the greater your chance is for successful breastfeeding and milk production.

The second type is called the Free Nipple Graft (FNG), which involves removing the nipple, and grafting it to a new location. This severs the blood and nerve supply to the nipple. Most women will lose sensation in the nipple and there is a dramatic impact to the ability to breastfeed. Most surgeons only use this if the patient's breasts are too large for the pedicle procedure. As you can imagine, disrupting the nipple and underlying tissue will likely result in minimal amounts of milk production.

Another procedure is a breast lift, also called a Mastoplexy. While this is technically not a breast reduction, it does rearrange tissue in certain areas of the breast. The procedure may involve removing tissue, replacing it with an implant and even liposuction in areas around the breast. Depending upon the extent of the breast lift, this may also impact supply. Many women will have this done because their breasts are different sizes. Therefore one breast might be more manipulated than the other. Less manipulation generally is better from a milk supply standpoint.

There are many stories of women successfully breastfeeding their baby after breast surgery. It's important to know the type of breast surgery you've had, so ask your surgeon if you are unsure. Each situation is different and it will be hard to predict what your outcomes might be. There is not one solution for every circumstance.

Many of you also have concerns about doing both breastfeeding and bottle-feeding. In fact, some of you are only interested in pumping and bottle-feeding. So let's look at the options out there for you.

Chapter 6: Can I still breastfeed if my baby takes a bottle?

Some women approach their breastfeeding experience wanting to do 'both breast and bottle' while others just want to pump and bottle feed. I have seen success with breastfeeding and bottle-feeding, what helps determine a more successful outcome usually depends upon when you introduce a bottle.

Many mothers are hesitant to begin bottles because they are afraid their baby will have nipple confusion. While this is a real concern, it generally is not a problem once you have breastfeeding well established. Introducing a bottle of breast milk after 2-3 weeks is a great way to get Dad or other family members involved with baby's feedings. Many mothers wonder if their baby will return to breastfeeding once they have had a bottle. I would like to put your mind at ease. The majority of babies will do just fine going back and forth between breastfeeding and bottle-feeding. The key is to wait until breastfeeding is going well, your milk supply is adequate and baby is gaining weight. Knowing your baby is back to their birth weight will put your mind at ease and most health care providers would like to see this at about two weeks of age.

Some mothers would like to only pump their breast milk and bottle-feed their baby. I have seen many women be successful with this method as well. There are some key elements to this being successful:

You must start pumping early; right after birth if possible

You must pump regularly; whenever the baby eats to establish a full milk supply

You must have a reliable double-electric pump

One of the biggest challenges for the 'pumping-only-to-bottle-feed' plan is keeping an adequate milk supply. The way the baby nurses and how often the baby nurses are the two driving forces for milk supply. A baby uses both sucking and compression, or up and down motions of their jaw when they are breastfeeding. The pump will only supply the sucking component. Unfortunately, there is no pump that provides a compression motion. When you are using only a pump for stimulation, there is the possibility of lower milk supply. Some women can compensate for this by using herbal supplements. We cover all our top herbal products later in this book. Most women find one or more of these suggestions to be helpful in maintaining an adequate milk supply.

Be sure to educate yourself and seek advice from a lactation consultant who works frequently with these situations. They see the outcomes and draw experience from mothers who have been successful. Finally, in Chapter Seven, I'll cover another subject where women have many questions regarding alcohol and medications.

Chapter 7: How do medications and alcohol affect the breast milk?

Some mothers need to take a medication or would like to enjoy a glass of wine at some point throughout their breastfeeding experience. "Can I have a glass of wine?" or "Can I take this medication?" are questions we hear on an almost daily basis. You have probably read or heard many different answers. I would like to tackle this from a medical standpoint with resources for you to lean on.

Most medications will not harm your baby. However to be safe, express your concerns to a lactation consultant for specific medications you may be taking. The guide that is frequently used by lactation consultants to research the effects and interactions of medications and breast milk is called '*Medications and Mother's Milk*' by Dr. Thomas Hale. This is the "bible" for medication interaction for most lactation consultants. I like this book because it lists medication information for both lactation and pregnancy. The author looks at many aspects of each drug such as the drug's half-life, molecular weight, and protein binding to list a few. Not many resources will provide such thorough research based answers. After all considerations and calculations, each medication is given a level of one through five. Number one is the safest and number five is a drug that should be avoided. The book also lists alternative medications that could be substituted as they offer more compatibility for breastfeeding. Be aware there are very few medications that are levels four and five. Knowing this information can help mothers and health care professionals make medication decisions based on accurate information.

Many women would like to enjoy an alcoholic beverage while they are nursing their baby. You should be aware that alcohol does pass through your breast milk. Here are some basic guidelines for you to follow:

- Alcohol goes rather quickly into breast milk, therefore it is best to breastfeed first, then enjoy your beverage.
- By the time you would nurse again the majority of the alcohol will be out of your milk. This varies based upon how much alcohol was consumed, of course.
- If you have a special occasion and are enjoying a 'few too many' and are feeling the effects of the alcohol, it is probably best to pump your breasts and discard the milk. This is a time to pump-and-dump as they say. Use previously pumped milk to feed your baby.

When you have to take a medication or wish to have a glass of wine, please don't feel you have to abandon breastfeeding. You can work breastfeeding around your life; don't work your life around breastfeeding. Remember all the good reasons you are choosing to breastfeed.

As you can see, there is really very little standing in the way between you and achieving your breastfeeding goals. Nursing your baby can be versatile and fit into your lifestyle very easily. I hope this book has helped you decide if breastfeeding is right for you. My aim is that you give breastfeeding a chance beyond the first few hours or even days of your baby's life. No one can provide this unique, species-specific liquid love for your baby.

My last bit of advice to you is this:

Look for accurate information as you make this decision. The more educated you are the more prepared you will be.

Get your support system in place. You may have to tap into them right away after the birth. Keep well-meaning people with negative advice at arms' length. They may love you and care about you and your baby, but they may not be giving you the answers you need or the support you are looking for.

Be patient with yourself and your baby. Trust yourself as the mother. No one knows your baby better than you do. After all, this relationship took 9 months to develop before you even laid eyes on each other! You already knew them before you met them.

Seek help whenever you feel the need. You may need to talk to a lactation consultant on a regular basis. You have to remember this is an ever-changing ride between a mother and her child. Getting help with your problems and answers to your questions can make the difference between a great experience and one you would like to forget.

I have experience in hospital based lactation programs and home care settings. I am a co-owner of a lactation business, "All About Lactation", which focuses on educating the health care professional. My colleague and I have helped thousands and thousands of women throughout their breastfeeding journey and have learned so much from them! I would like to pass all this knowledge on to you. I have no doubt this book can help make your breastfeeding experience everything you want and more. Everyone's journey is different; I can't promise you a problem-free ride. But I can promise you solid answers with evidence-based solutions. The best way to be prepared is to educate yourself. Don't wait until you have problems right on your door step, or when you have a baby who isn't gaining weight or is inconsolable at two in the morning. Light your path, be prepared and look for solutions. My goal is to help you! I want you to look back on this experience with nothing but happiness and joy knowing your gave your baby the best you!

Chapter 8: What's a Midwife, Doula or Lactation Consultant?

Since you've become pregnant you are likely talking to other mothers, health care providers and searching the web for some guidance and answers. New terms like "Midwives", "Doulas" and "Lactation Consultants" are likely popping up everywhere. But what do they mean and should you consider using some of their services?

A midwife or CNM (Certified Nurse Midwife) is a certified health care professional with a Master's Degree, who provides care to women during their pregnancy, labor, birth and during the postpartum period; the time right after delivery. They also have training in caring for your newborn and may even provide assistance with breastfeeding. They specialize in the delivery of women with low-risk pregnancies and are trained with the principle to "do not intervene unless necessary". Overall, midwives offer lower costs, less intervention, less mortality and morbidity due to fewer interventions, and their patients undergo fewer recovery complications.

A doula is known as a labor coach. They are typically non-medically trained women who have certifications and special training in labor and delivery. The primary goal of the doula is to help the mother feel safe by seeing her though her labor, and providing comfort and support. They assist a woman before, during and after her delivery. A doula may offer coaching support through the rough spots of labor and help you focus. The assistance of a doula during labor has been associated with improved outcomes for both mother and baby. There is research to support the benefits of having a doula. These benefits include: experiencing a shorter delivery, having less chance of a caesarean section and receiving a lesser amount of medication. Getting this support can provide a satisfying birth for both Mom and her partner. You need to feel especially comfortable with this person, as they will be very involved with you during this intimate moment of birth.

Some of you have never heard of a Lactation Consultant or you but don't know exactly how they might fit into the equation. There are a few different types of lactation assistance, which may have initials behind their name like, CLE, CLC and IBCLC. Although these letters or credentials may look similar, there is a difference.

A Certified Lactation Educator or CLE is not a lactation consultant. They are qualified to support and educate the public on breastfeeding related issues. The education they receive does not qualify them to give out medical advice, diagnose medical conditions for mom or baby, or prescribe treatment or medication. They may work as a WIC (Women Infant's and Children) peer counselors, a breast pump technician, teach breastfeeding classes or lead a breastfeeding support group.

Another credential in lactation is a CLC, or a Certified Lactation Counselor. Having a CLC certification means this person has received training and competency verification in breastfeeding and lactation support. The CLC works in partnership with other health care professionals to make referrals and recommendations. They may also work in the community to help increase breastfeeding rates, teach classes and assist mothers in nursing for a longer period of time. They work in hospitals, community facilities, physician or midwife offices, or they may be in private practice.

An IBCLC is someone who is credentialed as an International Board Certified Lactation Consultant. This credential identifies a knowledgeable and experienced member of the maternal-child health care team. It is the only international credentialing and is recognized all over the world. Most IBCLCs are Registered Nurses, however, they may also be dietitians, physicians or midwives. IBCLC's use a problem solving approach to the care they provide while using evidence-based research. They have experience with the more difficult lactation situations and scenarios. There are professional standards for IBCLCs to follow and they must renew their certification every 5 years by continuing education or re-examination.

Now that these different roles have been explained, you can determine how they may fit into your overall plan. You will find that interviewing these people will be quite helpful when searching for the right fit. Don't be shy, these professionals are accustomed to this approach and want to be a good fit as much as you do. I've discussed options of people who might help you along your pregnancy and delivery path; now let's tackle where you might deliver.

Chapter 9: What should I look for when choosing a hospital?

Once again you may find when doing your research that there are a lot of terms and acronyms out there. The medical world can be an overwhelming place if you don't "speak the language" or know the services available. So let's look at which services and features of a hospital or birthing center might benefit you. This will likely guide you to a comfortable decision.

A Baby Friendly Hospital Initiative (BFHI) is a worldwide program of UNICEF and The World Health Organization (WHO) launched in 1991. The main goal of Baby Friendly Hospital Initiative is to ensure that all facilities where mothers deliver support breastfeeding. There are 10 specific steps that hospitals or birthing centers need to implement in order to achieve Baby Friendly status. The process is controlled by global criteria that can be applied to maternity care in virtually every country. Currently in the United States, approximately 5% of all hospitals have the Baby Friendly Hospital Certification, in contrast, Sweden's hospitals are 100% Baby-Friendly. Since this initiative has begun, 134 countries have been awarded Baby-Friendly status. In areas where Baby-Friendly status has been achieved, more mothers breastfeed and child health improvements are seen. For a complete listing of all facilities that have a Baby Friendly distinction, please visit the UNICEF website at www.unicef.org/programme/breastfeeding/assets/statusbfhi.pdf.

The IBCLC Care Award is a special recognition given to Hospital-Based Facilities and Community-Based Agencies that staff IBCLCs as part of their care team. To become eligible, the facility must have current

IBCLCs on staff, have a professional lactation support program, which is available 5-7 days per week, complete breastfeeding training to all staff, and have projects in place that promote and support breastfeeding. Chosen facilities have a certificate of recognition and are listed in the IBCLC Care Directory beginning January of each year. To access this program, you can visit their website at www.IBCLCcare.org.

Some of you may give birth to a premature or sick baby. Even though you didn't plan for this, it will be the time you rely on a Special Care Nursery (SCN) or Neonatal Intensive Care Unit (NICU). The skill and knowledge of the staff in these units will be invaluable to you as they care for, and teach you to care for your special baby.

There are three different levels of care a hospital provides for your baby. Be aware not all hospitals have SCN or NICU capabilities at their facilities. The Normal Newborn Nursery is considered a Level 1; it cares for healthy term babies.

A SCN is considered a Level 2 nursery where the care provided is intermediate. These infants may need special therapy or feedings that may prevent them from going home with their families. This may include a 35-37 week baby who is near-term, a jaundice baby who needs bilirubin lights or a baby who just needs to grow bigger before going home.

Finally, a Level 3 Nursery, or NICU, treats newborns needing high technology such as ventilators, intravenous therapy or feeding tubes. This nursery cares for just about all premature newborns, from 23-35 weeks gestation. There may be other newborns here, with chromosomal abnormalities or traumatic births. When deciding where to deliver, you should consider the hospitals ability to care for you and your baby if special care or intensive care are needed.

Hopefully this helps guide you to a comfortable decision. Most hospitals and birthing centers offer tours for you to view the facilities and learn about their services. You can learn about their services on their websites as well. The topic of human donor milk may be unfamiliar to some of you. For many of you this topic may raise some questions, which is great, because I have the answers!

Chapter 10: What is donor milk and is it safe?

This topic often raises questions along with many emotions; as well it should. In this day and age of transmittable diseases, is this really a safe solution? After all, we're talking about your baby's health and well being! Is this really a good option for your child and is it a safe option? The answer is yes. It's beneficial to have all the knowledge available about donor milk; this will help you decide if using donor breast milk is right for you and your baby.

Your breast milk is considered the "Gold Standard" of food for you baby. However, under certain circumstances your milk may not be readily available. The next "best food" for your baby is human donor milk. Donor milk is breast milk that is donated by other mothers who produce extra milk to help feed babies across the country. The donor mothers are not paid by the milk bank, so they do this purely out of love and concern for other children. Currently there are 13 existing milk banks across North America. There are also several more milk banks in the development process. A milk bank tests, processes and distributes the milk to hospitals and birthing centers. The mothers and their milk go through a very strict screening and testing process. Here are the steps involved:

- Telephone interview with the potential donating mother
- Written application filled out by the mother
- Mother has blood drawn and tested for a variety of illnesses
- Milk is collected and tested
- The milk is pasteurized by heating to 145 degrees for 30 minutes.

- Pasteurization reduces pathogens likely to cause disease.
- The milk is then retested for bacteria after pasteurizing
- Milk is frozen for distribution

This gives you an idea of the rigorous processing involved. Donated breast milk is actually screened more closely than blood donation. For more information about donor milk please visit www.hmbana.org.

Does your potential facility have donor milk available if your baby requires it? This would be one question to ask when you are making the choice of the facility for your delivery. Hospitals and birthing centers purchase donated milk. Most milk banks charge $4.50 per ounce to pay for the extensive processing and distribution. Some insurance companies will pay for this if the baby's condition requires it and the physician orders the milk. If there is not insurance reimbursement to the facility, the facility usually pays for the cost of the milk. A facility concerned for you and has your baby's best interests will have donor milk available. By having donor milk available, they are showing their commitment to helping the breastfeeding process and desire to have the best outcome for all their babies.

Once you have all the information about the donor milk process and the benefits, it's not such a daunting concept. It's wise to be prepared and educated about using human donor milk. You will need to be at ease with this option if you are delivering at a facility where they offer donor milk. Now that you are informed about human donor milk, let's talk about breast pumps. How do you know which pump is right for you? This next chapter will help you decide.

Chapter 11: What should I look for when choosing a breast pump?

Choosing a pump that best fits your personal needs can be tricky. Every mom has a different plan, need and budget in mind.

Hospital-grade pumps are heavy-duty efficient pumps that have a rapid suck and release cycle. They are used by hospitals, clinics and lactation rooms for employees to pump while at work. This type of pump is designed to be a multi-user pump, since many people can use the same breast pump. Each person however needs their personal pumping kit, which contains all the plastic pieces that collect the milk. This, like most pumps, is a double electric pump. This means you can remove milk from both breasts at the same time. These pumps are high quality and typically too expensive to own as your personal pump. They range in cost from $700-$2,500 per pump. However, these pumps can be rented on a monthly basis. Some find they want or need the quality and efficiency of a hospital-grade pump and renting will provide them with this option less expensively.

The next option is a personal use double electric pump. These are affordable, portable and convenient for women who have an established milk supply. Designed for a single user, these pumps are not meant for sharing. Again, this double electric pump is designed to pump both breasts at the same time. This is essential when a woman is relying on a pump to help keep up her supply. Not only will double pumping save you time, it stimulates better than a single pump. If you are planning to use your pump daily, you will likely need a double pump to keep an adequate milk supply. The cost of this type of pump ranges from $250-$350.

Another option would be a less expensive electric or battery operated breast pump. These are designed for short term or occasional use. They generally allow for one-sided pumping, therefore taking more time. The motor often does not last as long as the more expensive models. If the pump is battery operated, the batteries will need replacing often. These pumps can range in price from $100-$200.

Lastly there is a manual pump. They typically require you to squeeze a lever or pump a piston to create the suction. They are designed to pump one breast at a time and may require both hands to use. Hand pumps are generally the most affordable and quiet of the pumps available. Some moms have trouble moving milk down when using a hand pump and find them rather tedious. If you are going to pump only rarely, maybe to leave milk for an evening out, this might work well for you. The price range for this breast pump is from $50-$100.

If you plan to return to work and pump, you may be using your pump for a full year or more and the price of a good pump will be well worth it. Remember while you are feeding breast milk to your baby, the cost savings of not purchasing alternative milk or formula will pay for the pump rather quickly. Don't try to get by cheaply, as you will get what you pay for. Never purchase a used personal breast pump. You do not know if the previous user's milk may have backed into the pump and bacteria will grow in the milk residue. When looking at breast pumps the advice and assistance of a lactation consultant is extremely valuable. They are often asked for breast pump advice and they are the ones that see the results of most pumps on the market.

There are many options out there so find the pump that will work best for your situation. If your goal is long-term nursing, invest in a good pump because it will likely keep you nursing/pumping longer. As we learned earlier, the longer you breastfeed the better for both you and your baby. Your choice of a breast pump will most likely impact your total breastfeeding experience. Also, pumping helps get your partner involved. We'll talk about that next.

Chapter 12: Is Daddy feeling left out?

Breastfeeding is a very intimate time between mom and baby. At times it may feel like there is no one else in the room but you and your baby. There is nothing in the world like it. Unfortunately, sometimes dads or partners feel left out and wonder how they're going to bond with their child. Babies do more than just eat; there's room for everyone to share in the joy!

Skin-to-skin care, sometimes called Kangaroo Mother Care, involves placing your baby's bare chest directly onto your bare chest, this is an activity dads love to do. There is growing research and evidence that skin-to-skin contact right after birth helps babies in many ways, including:

- Calming and relaxing both mother and baby
- Helps baby to stabilize their temperature and blood sugars
- Helps to regulate baby's heart rate and breathing patterns
- Allows baby to be colonized by mother's 'friendly' bacteria, not that of a infant warmer or incubator
- Stimulates baby's feeding behavior which teaches mother baby's feeding cues immediately
- Stimulates the release of hormones that support breastfeeding
- Encourages baby to cry less
- Promotes baby's ability to exclusively breastfeed longer

These are just a few of the benefits of skin-to-skin care. It is also documented that 20 minutes of skin-to-skin will reduce cortisol levels, which are stress hormones, in the mother by 48% and in baby by 67%. High levels of cortisol interfere with baby's ability to organize and breastfeed. This is very important to a baby when they are learning the activity of breastfeeding. When a baby is taken out of their natural habitat, they show signs of being under stress. Skin-to-skin can eliminate this unnecessary stress.

When your baby is born, If possible, I recommend that you stay skin-to-skin with your baby until the two of you have had a good first breastfeeding session. Do not interrupt this time for other things such as weighing, measuring or giving a shot for instance. Let the staff or midwife know your wishes. This time is precious and significant in your baby's life. Babies that have a good first feeding in the first 1-2 hours following birth have more successful feedings later on.

All these benefits are even more important if your baby is born prematurely or ill. Regular skin-to-skin contact helps these babies become more stable, to maintain their own body temperature, to grow and develop more quickly, to develop a stronger ability to fight infection and to be discharged from the hospital sooner. After all, isn't that your ultimate goal, getting a healthy baby home as soon as possible?

Now, getting back to the Dads: Dad and Partner are also encouraged to practice regular skin-to-skin with their baby. The benefits to baby aren't exclusively given by mom. So share the activity, participate in skin-to-skin and reap some of the fun! What a wonderful process, relax and snuggle with your baby!

There are other baby cares that need to be done and these can all be shared. In fact, it will be good to share them so mom doesn't feel overwhelmed and can get some much needed rest. Some may think the role of the dad or partner is minor, yet studies show a support person plays a very critical role in the success of breastfeeding. Study after study supports the theory that breastfeeding longevity and success all hinge on the breastfeeding mother's support system.

Dads and partners should do plenty of skin-to-skin as mentioned above. Other baby cares will include bathing, changing diapers and burping, to name a few. These all need to be done and when you participate in these cares your baby will get to know your voice, touch and scent. These things are all very important for the bonding process. Let them fall asleep while doing skin-to-skin on your chest. Your baby will make the connection that you too can provide comfort, security and love. This will also free up mom for some extra rest periods she will likely need during the first few weeks.

Many times dads or partners of breastfed babies are anxious to be involved with feeding their new baby. This usually means giving the baby a bottle. The mechanics of breastfeeding and bottle-feeding are very different and introducing a bottle too early may be confusing for your baby. When a baby breastfeeds, their tongue and jaws work together in a rhythmic motion as they cup their tongue under the areola of the breast, and compress the nipple between the tongue and the roof of their mouth. When a baby drinks from a bottle, the milk often comes out rather quickly. They need to use their tongue to block the flow of milk to prevent them from choking. When the breast has a let down, it is often with a slower trickle allowing the baby to have control over the feeding. While most babies can eventually shift easily between breast and bottle, here are a few suggestions for a smoother transition:

- Wait until Mom's milk is in fully
- See that Baby is back to birth weight, which is usually around 2 weeks
- Wait until breastfeeding is well established
- Wait until there are no concerns with Mother or Baby, i.e. sore nipples, difficulty latching
- Use a slow flow nipple to avoid the gulping type of defensive sucking that is needed with the faster flowing nipples

You will likely have greater success transitioning to bottles and continuing to breastfeed if your follow these guidelines. Having your partner interact with baby and being involved with their care is very important to the development of your child. Time should be set aside for just those two. Mom will appreciate the break and support. But the support shouldn't stop here. The wider the circle the more successful you will experience.

Chapter 13: Is your support system in place?

Getting your support team in place before you deliver will make the transition go smoothly. After delivery most people have an adjustment period while getting used to their new role and all the responsibility it brings. You will be faced with some new challenges. If you can divide your new tasks and share them as a team it will help the process along.

Many years ago people lived in a village with their relatives as their support system right at hand. Today this is usually not the case. The 21st century mother may need to assemble her support team. That team and who is on it, becomes the key to your success. Your support team may consist of parents, in-laws, friends, neighbors and even coworkers. Whoever you choose on your team, be sure they all have one thing in common; that they support you and your breastfeeding efforts. If your in-law is going to say, "Oh, just one bottle of formula won't hurt" or your mother says "I formula fed you and you're just fine." perhaps they shouldn't be asked to be on your team. You need cheerleaders! These are people who can give you confidence and hold you up during a tough moment. You need someone who understands your goals and will do whatever they can to help you achieve those goals. Usually other women who have breast-fed are good "go-to" people and can offer good advice. A lactation consultant is a wise choice to have on your team. Have her phone number close by.

Be sure your family practice doctor or pediatrician also supports your decision to breastfeed. Some may give poor advice and can put your breastfeeding efforts to a halt! Others can turn a bad situation around and make it better. Ask your baby's doctor how they feel about breastfeeding. This may help and guide you to someone who would be the most helpful to you. Find a doctor who is supportive and can help you have a positive experience. Some clinics even have lactation assistance right at their clinic.

Many women find support with other breastfeeding women. Find a Le Leche League support group near you. These groups are full of women who have your same goals in mind. They can guide you and become the cheerleader you need to succeed. Some local hospitals or clinics may also provide a breastfeeding support group. Perhaps there is one at your work place or at a local church. This is an option worth verifying.

Unfortunately, stress and fatigue can become part of being a new parent. Between keeping up with the night feedings and experiencing shorter sleep cycles, you may become fatigued. It is important for your support team to help minimize your stress and help you get the extra rest your body needs. Attempting to get more sleep may require you to nap when your baby naps. This is not a time to clean the house, answer your email or do some cooking. It's a time to rest. Go to bed a little earlier or ask someone to watch your baby while you catch up on some needed rest.

Some stress relievers may help your overall health as well; eat right, get some extra rest, talk to others about your stressors, keep a journal to help you understand what is stressful in your life, and become physically active. All these may help decrease the stress, as your life seems to have changed overnight.

Having realistic expectations and having your support system in place are all important aspects to work on while you are pregnant. When people ask what they can do for you...tell them! Give them a list such as; 'help with the laundry', 'go grocery shopping', 'look after the baby while I take a nap', 'bring dinner'. If you have trouble asking for or accepting help, it will be in your best interest to be open minded to the idea. It might be something very small, but it is something you can cross off your list and keep the focus on you and your baby.

Once you settle in to your new role and life becomes a bit more predictable, it will be time to start thinking about becoming intimate again.

Some of you might feel like that is "light years away" but this too will come sooner than you think. So what are the best options for a breast-feeding mother?

Chapter 14: What type of birth control is best when I'm breastfeeding?

Yes, before you know it your health care provider will be asking you what type of birth control you want to use. This may be the farthest thing from your mind. It certainly is for many new moms. My sister revealed that when her doctor told her no intercourse for 4-6 weeks, she added the weeks together and told her husband, "no sex for 10 weeks!" You might feel like taking her advice. However, knowing which birth control choice is best for you will be determined by the impact it has on your short and long term nursing goals. Some options are better than others. Let's take a look at them.

Depo-Provera is a branded progestin-only contraceptive. This is a drug that is injected into a large muscle group, such as your buttock or arm every 3 months. It provides instant protection. Most literature suggests delaying the injection until six weeks postpartum. When using progestin, many women experience a decrease in milk production especially when the hormone is given in the first few days after delivery. If you would like this option of birth control, it is best to wait until your six week check up and be sure you have a full milk supply.

The birth control pill includes a combination of estrogen and progestin that is taken by mouth every day. This combination birth control pill is not recommended for breastfeeding women. The estrogen portion of the pill will most likely produce a decrease in milk supply. In fact, many women actually lose their milk in a short period of time.

There is another option for those wanting to take the pill. The mini pill is a progestin only pill that does not contain any estrogen. This pill prevents ovulation and causes thickening of the cervical mucous thereby decreasing sperm penetration. This is a much better option for women wanting an oral contraceptive. It's best if you wait until you have a full milk supply before beginning the mini pill. If you are struggling at all with milk supply, it's best if you to use another method.

Barrier methods have been used for centuries. These provide birth control without the use of hormones, which may decrease your supply. The most common barrier methods are condoms, diaphragms or IUDs. All are great options and you can get fitted for a diaphragm at your six week check up.

Breastfeeding is a natural way to space your children and provide all the birth control you may need. Breastfeeding can suppress ovulation from occurring. When you breastfeed, the hormone prolactin suppresses the release of hormones that can cause the eggs to mature and the uterine lining to prepare for the eggs arrival. This is why nursing mothers usually do not get a period while they are exclusively breastfeeding. This method can be 98% effective; providing you follow some simple practices:

Nurse your baby frequently, every 2-3 hours during the daytime. This will help keep prolactin high and fertility hormones low.

Night nursing is a very effective way to keep ovulation away. Fertility hormones tend to be highest during the nighttime hours, therefore night feedings may keep these hormones in balance.

Avoid supplemental bottles. Introducing formula will decrease the milk making hormone

Delay introducing solids until baby is 6 months old. You will likely notice your baby will decrease the number of nursing sessions once you begin solids.

Studies have shown that by following these four simple guidelines, women will average a 14 month delay before their period returns. If your periods have returned you can assume that breastfeeding is no longer a reliable method of birth control.

Your birth control choices are important to your overall breastfeeding goals. I wanted to be sure you had some solid answers so you can choose wisely. Being prepared on the topics discussed can help you make your best decisions. You want to set yourself up to be as successful as possible. Every woman has breastfeeding dreams they want to see come true. You deserve that realization! Stay focused on the prize and I'll continue to guide you through the steps.

Chapter 15: How do I get off to a great start?

Now that your baby has arrived, parenting begins immediately. There are some key first steps to take as you begin. You are now getting to know this new little person you have created and provided with life. No matter what the setting was for this birth; a hospital, birthing center, your home or even in a car; the actions are the same. Let your maternal instincts take over and remember this time of bonding with your baby forever.

As long as you and your baby are feeling fine, it is best to initiate skin-to-skin right away after baby is born. This is the most alert time for baby; the first 2 hours of life, so take advantage of this moment. After their initial crying stage to expand their lungs, babies enter a relaxation stage. This is followed by an active alert state where their eyes are open and they have head movements and mouth activity. They may crawl up your body and reach toward your breast and seek out the nipple. They are familiarizing themselves with the "outside" of you. Once they find your nipple they will begin suckling and beginning their first of many more feedings to come. They will self-attach within an hour of birth. After their first feeding they will be exhausted and enter a restful sleep. This feeding is very important to the success of breastfeeding because imprinting is occurring. Imprinting is a rapid learning process that establishes a behavior pattern and recognition. In effect baby will remember the success of this first feeding and attempt to pattern other feedings after that one. This imprinting almost always leads to improved breastfeeding during the first several days. So feed early and feed often.

Skin-to-skin was addressed earlier, but it's so important it deserves to be revisited. Skin-to-skin has been defined as early and exclusive time for mother and baby to bond and connect. It meets the needs of both of you emotionally, physically and psychologically. When a baby is left with their mother right after birth, Mother is assisting baby to stabilize their body functions and vital signs. Your baby is being comforted by your voice, heartbeat, smell, body heat and your touch. No one can provide this level of comfort but you. Take advantage of this special time, both of you will need this time right after birth. It is almost magical!

In addition, spend as much time as possible doing skin-to-skin during the first few days. This helps your baby continue to stabilize their body functions as they begin their life. Research has found that providing skin-to-skin to your baby will improve their long-term emotional stability. They will have successful breastfeeding with a longer duration. You are learning your baby's hunger signs while baby has greater access to their food. In addition, developmental pathways to the brain grow in a calm tranquil setting, as opposed to an atmosphere influenced by stress and confusion. After all, the primary bond between a mother and a child is the basis on which all subsequent relationships are built. It's not a tough assignment; all you need to do is snuggle and touch your baby as much as possible.

What about the times when it's not possible for the mother to do skin-to-skin? This is where Dad comes in. In fact, dads and partners should do skin-to-skin their bonding should also begin as soon as possible. Some parents take this job very seriously. The story below will define this further:

A mother had a rough delivery followed by a postpartum hemorrhage. She had lost so much blood; she had to get a blood transfusion. The dad felt so helpless as he watched the blood going into his wife and his baby crying in the bassinet. I told him the best thing he could do for his baby was to do skin-to-skin. I explained the process to him and went out of their hospital room to get a warm blanket. I was about 10 feet down the hall when I realized I forgot to ask him a question. When I returned seconds later I found him standing in the middle of the room in nothing but his boxers holding his naked baby against his chest! I was a little surprised at the speed of his efforts, however it was very sweet to see him spring into action so quickly. I got them settled in with the warm blanket and they both relaxed. I did mention to him that he could keep his pants on!

Another reason to breastfeed early and often is related to the hormone prolactin. Prolactin is the hormone responsible for milk production and breast tissue growth to prepare the breasts for producing milk. Prolactin levels are lower during the first trimester of your pregnancy where they measure approximately 20 ng/L. These levels gradually increase until your third trimester when they measure 100+ ng/L. After delivery of the placenta, there is a sharp rise in prolactin levels. It's your body's way of saying "we don't need estrogen and progesterone any more...baby is here!" These levels have been measured to be 300-400 ng/L. This is the perfect time to give your body the message "Yes, we are breastfeeding!" Prolactin levels rise and fall in proportion to the frequency, intensity and duration of nipple stimulation. So putting baby to the breast early gives you the benefit of these hormones. As higher levels are reached it typically means higher milk production. After 7+ days prolactin levels have already dropped to around 100 ng/L. Therefore, laying the foundation for a full milk supply begins right away. Take advantage of this first week while your hormones are high and highly responsive.

You can appreciate how important those first few hours of life are to the new baby. There are many influences taking place during this time of transition. Imprinting is extremely important. The benefits of skin-to-skin continue, the more research being done, more benefits are discovered. After delivery your hormones are primed and ready to go into action, take advantage of this time to help lay the groundwork for a full milk supply.

Another aspect to getting off to a good start, is positioning your baby at the breast. Which position(s) offer more success than others? Let's find out what might be right for you.

Chapter 16: What are the best positions for successful breastfeeding?

This time of getting to know your baby is a wonderful moment in your life. Yes, breastfeeding is a natural behavior, but at first it may not seem so natural. Learning how to support, hold and feed your baby comfortably will take patience and practice. Finding the correct position(s) for you and your baby will likely be trial and error. Sometimes what has worked in the past will work just fine for subsequent children; however this isn't always the case, as no two babies are the same. I will describe a variety of positions, why they might be good for you, and under which circumstances they might work best. I want to emphasize that all positions begin with mom and baby comfortable and baby fully awake, with a wide open mouth and ready to nurse.

The cradle hold is the most "classic" position, which calls for you to cradle the top of your baby's head within the crook of your arm. Have a comfortable chair with armrests, plenty of pillows and possibly a footstool or coffee table to put up your feet. Place a pillow on your lap, position baby across your lap while they are lying on their side. Be sure their tummy is touching your tummy and they are directly facing you. Tuck their lower arm under your own arm so baby can be close to you. You don't want their tummy or face to be facing upwards, as this is an awkward position for anyone to drink. If the baby is nursing on your left breast, their head is in the crook of your left arm. Your left arm and hand supports their back, neck and perhaps their bottom, while your right hand supports your breast. The positions are reversed when the baby is nursing on your right breast. This position works best for full term babies who have not experienced a traumatic delivery. Mother's who deliver by cesarean section often find this position places extra stress on a tender abdomen. This position is slightly more difficult, as you are first learning.

The cross-cradle or crossover position is slightly different from the cradle position in that you don't hold your baby's head in the crook of your arm. Instead, you are providing support with your hand around the base of the neck and lower portion of the head. If you are nursing on your left breast, you use your left hand to support the breast and your right hand and arm support the baby's back, neck and bottom. Baby is still facing you and both of you are still tummy-to-tummy. This is a great position in the beginning while you are both learning. This works well for small babies, premature babies or those having difficulty latching on. This is considered a more direct position for the baby making it easier for them to latch. You are providing guidance to the breast, not pushing the baby's head into the breast.

Side-lying position is used when you are lying in bed on your side. At first you may need to have your partner assist you and will likely need more pillows for support. Be sure your back, neck and baby are all supported. Have your baby face you, again tummy-to-tummy. If you are lying on your left side bring baby in closely with your right hand and arm. Having someone else tuck baby in for the latch will be very helpful. Once baby is latched, placing a pillow against their back will give them the support while allowing you to be more relaxed. This position is best if you have had a cesarean birth or a difficult vaginal birth where sitting up is uncomfortable. Sometimes women with larger breasts also find this position works well. This position may take a bit more practice, so be patient with yourself.

Lastly, the Clutch or Football Hold may be right for you. This is done by placing your baby under your arm like a football or purse. If baby is nursing on your left side, baby is tucked under your left arm and you are holding and guiding your baby with your left hand and arm. Be sure to have a pillow under your arm so baby is primarily resting on the pillow. Your right hand will be supporting your left breast for an easier latch.

Your left arm is guiding baby in for a latch. Be careful you are not holding the entire weight of the baby on your arms; baby's weight is mainly on the pillow. Some women tense up and raise their shoulders while they are feeding the baby. Try to relax and let the pillow carry the load, or you may find you have sore shoulders when you are finished. This football hold works well if your breasts are larger, as it lets you better see your baby and know when their mouth is ready for the latch. This is also nice if you have had a Cesarean delivery, as it keeps the weight of the baby off your abdomen. Smaller babies also do well with this position because it allows you to guide them more directly to your nipple. Babies that seem to be somewhat disorganized will also do well in this position. Placing baby into a familiar 'tucked' position will remind them of how they were inside of you sucking on fingers and toes. This may help them become more organized as they return to a well-known position. Lastly, women with flatter nipples have more success using the clutch position because their field of vision is greater to see best opportunity for latching.

Finding a position or two that work well for both of you may come easy or it might take a few tries. Having someone help you makes this discovery easier than going it alone. That's why other people are there to help, to make it easier for you! Whether it is your partner, a nurse, midwife, doula, sister or friend, they all want you to succeed. Sometimes you may feel like it takes two sets of hands to latch one little baby. You are not alone, most new mothers feel this way. It's all part of getting to know your baby. Knowing that you have a good latch is another concern most moms have. There are some quick and easy tips to help and guide you.

Chapter 17: How do I know if I have a good latch?

Having someone tell you your baby has a good latch is encouraging; however actually knowing this for yourself is even better. You will likely question this for some of your early latches. Moms are constantly asking nurses and their health care providers, "Is this a good latch?" and, "Does this look right to you?" This is one way to get the feedback you need, the problem is they won't be available forever. Assessing a latch is something you will need to learn yourself. So let's spend this chapter looking at this important part of breastfeeding so you can answer that question for yourself.

If there were one myth I could stop moms from fearing, it would have to be "breastfeeding hurts". Breastfeeding should not hurt or be painful, at least within some specific guidelines I will describe. As mentioned previously, breastfeeding may take a little practice. Here are three questions to ask yourself while your baby is breastfeeding that will help you know if you have a good latch.

#1 - Is your pain level a three or under when baby is nursing? On a pain scale of 0-10 with 0 being no pain and a 10 being the worst pain you know: perhaps labor pain; you should have a pain level of three or under. Minimal discomfort is a normal aspect of breastfeeding. Initially you may have 30 seconds or so of pain that is greater than a three. This is usually caused by the nipple and areola being pulled into baby's mouth. Sometimes it may take a few seconds for baby to get 'organized' and into a good sucking rhythm. However, beyond the first several seconds, your pain level should be a three or under.

#2 - Is your baby productively nursing? Babies will suck in a productive or nutritive pattern or in a non-productive or non-nutritive pattern. With the productive pattern you will see large jaw movements, activity and motion by the ears and temple muscles. You will hear a quiet "K" sound now and again. This is the sound they make when they are swallowing. In the beginning days of breastfeeding, you may only hear swallows every 7-10 sucks. Be assured this is normal. Swallows will be heard more often in the next few days as your supply increases. You will also feel a slight tugging and pulling when baby is nursing productively.

When a baby is in a non-productive nursing pattern you will likely feel more biting and chewing, which will cause your pain level to be greater than three. Your baby will have smaller jaw movements and little to no temple muscle involvement if nursing is in a non-productive pattern.

#3 - Is the shape of your nipple round when the feeding is finished? Your nipple should still look round after a feeding. If the nipple is coming out of the baby's mouth looking flat, creased, pinched or shaped like a new tube of lipstick, your baby wasn't on deeply enough. When beginning the feeding, baby should have a wide open mouth, like they are yawning or going to bite an apple.

To examine the structure of the mouth, you can run your tongue across the roof of your own mouth; you will feel the ridge where the roof becomes softer. This is the edge of your soft palate. This placement protects your nipple from baby's strong tongue muscle and from the firmness of the hard palate. Your baby should bring the tip of your nipple back to the soft palate. The more breast tissue the baby draws into their mouth, the more comfortable it is for you. Baby can lengthen your nipple to nearly 3 times the normal resting length while nursing.

If the answer to any of these three questions is "No", you need to get some help with latching. Don't be afraid to ask for assistance from nurses, your health care provider and especially from a lactation consultant. Getting help sooner rather than later can make a big difference in your overall experience.

I suggest you ask yourself these three questions whenever you are latching your baby to the breast. These questions will guide you to feel more comfortable and confident about breastfeeding.

There is also another sign to help you know your baby is doing well and getting your breast milk. Are you experiencing uterine cramping? Remember the hormone oxytocin? This hormone is released during breastfeeding to contract the lobes and ducts in your breast. Here is a little anatomy lesson: The inside of your breast is made up of about 15-20 lobes. Each lobe has many smaller lobules, which end in dozens of smaller bulbs that produce milk. These lobes and lobules are linked together by small tubes called ducts. When the baby sucks, triggering the release of the hormone oxytocin, it causes contractions in both your breast ducts and your uterus. You may feel your uterus contracting during the early days of breastfeeding, because the muscles in your uterus react to the oxytocin. In the early days of breastfeeding, this contracting is a good sign that baby is nursing well and getting milk while breastfeeding.

There are other signs you should be watching for to help you feel confident things are going well. Ask yourself "Is your baby satisfied after nursing?" They should either fall deeply asleep or have quiet awake time after nursing. Some babies may continue to root after you take them off the breast. Try to nurse them a little longer, perhaps going to the first side again. They may need to be "topped off". To keep them awake, stimulate them by rubbing their back, tickling their feet or gently blowing on their face. If they fall asleep or begin nursing in a non-productive pattern when you offer the breast for a second time, they are likely done breastfeeding. Nursing is a very cozy experience, where babies often become too comfortable. Keep them busy and focused on breastfeeding.

Keep track of all feedings, wet and dirty diapers until you know breastfeeding is going well and your baby is gaining weight. Your health care provider will likely ask, at their first check-up, how often baby is eating and how many diapers you are changing. Baby will need to have frequent weight checks until you know they are doing well and have established a good pattern of weight gain. After you deliver, hospitals and birthing centers will weigh your baby daily to be sure they aren't loosing too much weight. All babies lose weight, but how much they lose is what's important. You don't want your baby to lose more than 10% of their birth weight. If your baby is at or near this weight loss, you and your baby should have a feeding plan started by a lactation consultant or a knowledgeable health care provider to help you turn things around. This is when the expertise of a lactation consultant will be vital. Your baby should be weighed 2-3 days after discharge from a hospital or birth center, or when they are 2-3 days of age after a home birth. Sometimes they may need daily weight checks until they have stabilized. As we know ladies, the scale doesn't lie! For the most accurate weights your baby should be weighed naked. Accurate weights are very important when assessing a newborn condition.

Now you have some tools and means to answer that daunting question, "Is this a good latch?" You also have the knowledge to get help if the answer to any of the questions is "No". In certain situations you may need some extra assistance. Some deliveries are more traumatic that others. This trauma or distress can leave either mom or baby (or both) in a situation that needs attention. Next let's tackle some of these stressful situations for both mom and baby and what you can do to positively impact breastfeeding.

Chapter 18: I had a rough delivery; what can I expect now?

Most women anticipate a few rough moments during their labor and delivery. Some of you have already experienced this with previous children. What can you do if a rough moment actually happens? Let's look at some of the more likely possibilities or situations and give you some answers that will actually help.

As previously mentioned, stressful situations can happen to either mom or baby. In some situations it can be both. Let's start with you, the mom.

A cesarean birth or C-section is a surgical procedure where an incision is made in the abdomen and uterus to deliver the baby. According to <u>Healthgrades 2012,</u> which trends women's health in American hospitals, "the percentage of C-section births has reached and all-time high of 34%." I would suggest you ask your doctor about their groups'

C-section delivery rate, as well as the rate recorded at the facility where you are planning your birth. Having abdominal surgery to deliver your baby means a slower and more risky recovery.

If you do have a C-section, you are still encouraged to spend quality time with your baby immediately. Skin-to-skin, breastfeeding and letting baby make that transition to life can still happen right with you. If you know you are delivering your baby this way, contact your hospital and be aware of what their policies and procedures are regarding C-section births. Most women can still breastfeed comfortably as mentioned previously. Stay on top of your pain, which too should ideally be a three or under on your pain scale of 0-10. Most hospitals provide pain medications that are safe and compatible with breastfeeding, since this is a concern for many mothers.

Some women may hemorrhage after delivery. A postpartum hemorrhage is defined as a significant amount of blood loss after delivery of a baby. There are a variety of reasons a hemorrhage might occur but the most common reason is called uterine atony. This is the inability of the uterus to contract as it attempts to return to its pre-pregnant state, which is about the size of your fist. As you can imagine, there is a great deal of contracting needed to return your uterus back to this size. As mentioned, breastfeeding will release the hormone Oxytocin, which naturally contracts the uterus; so get that baby nursing right after delivery! Women who have experienced a postpartum hemorrhage usually develop low hemoglobin. Hemoglobin (abbreviated Hgb) is the iron and oxygen-transporting component in red blood cells. Hgb carries oxygen from the lungs, and circulates it where it is used by the body. Having a low Hbg usually means you tire easily, are pale and may have a delay in milk production.

Some vaginal deliveries can leave you with a sore bottom, possible hemorrhoids and a large repair. You may have some difficulty moving around. Again, stay on top of the pain. Many women find soaking in a tub or sitz bath is helpful and provides good relief. You can apply creams or sprays to your bottom, as many of them are designed to decrease the swelling and encourage healing. When you are breastfeeding, find a position where you are most comfortable. There is no need to change positions once you find one that works well for the two of you. Many women find an inflatable ring or donut helpful when sitting, while others will use a pillow for comfortable sitting. It is helpful if you tighten your gluteus muscles as you sit down, to prevent painful spreading when you sit down.

There is also potential trauma for baby as well. They have to go through quite a bit as they enter their new world. Their to do list becomes rather large once they are born. It was pretty much a free-ride inside of you, now their little bodies have to step up to the plate. They have to breathe on their own, circulate their blood, and manage their own heart, body temperature, and blood sugars to name a few tasks. No wonder they are tired! But all this intensifies if your baby has had added trauma to the normal functions they are now responsible for. Head trauma may exist if you had a particularly difficult delivery. Sometimes forceps or vacuum extraction is needed to get your baby delivered quickly and safely. Traumatic births may delay breastfeeding. Your baby is learning a new task and they might not be up for the challenge right away. They may be sleepier, need more time adjusting or have a harder time organizing the entire process of breastfeeding. They have to learn the pattern of suck-swallow-breath and this may not come easily when head trauma is involved. It's important to do as much skin-to-skin as possible. This will help your little one adjust and significantly decrease their stress, allowing them to be more organized with the breastfeeding process.

The good news is that transitioning doesn't last forever. Your baby will wake up and be ready to learn breastfeeding as part of their natural survival instincts. If there is a delay in breastfeeding, it will be helpful to use a breast pump. Pumping provides a way to get some of your breast milk to your baby and provide you with some needed stimulation. Most care givers feel your baby should have a good feeding within 8-12 hours of birth, others feel babies could go a bit longer. Ask for help and direction from your health care providers and a lactation consultant. As the trauma lessens and baby's swelling decreases, their interest in breastfeeding will return, with pumping or supplementing no longer needed.

Your baby may experience difficulty maintaining their blood sugar or their body temperature. Again, the best way to warm up a baby is to do skin-to-skin. Your breasts have the ability to increase in temperature two degrees in two minutes to warm your baby. Nothing is more effective than this! So before someone puts your baby back under an infant warmer, try skin-to-skin with a warm blanket over both of you. It works like a charm and this way baby can stay right with you which is less stressful for both. Skin-to-skin also helps them adjust their blood sugars. Sometimes baby's blood sugars are too low and they need to increase this as soon as possible. The best thing to do is breastfeed. If your baby is too sleepy to nurse effectively, you should use a breast pump or manually express some colostrum for your baby. This will provide the instant glucose or sugar they need.

If you were heavily medicated during your delivery, this may delay effective breastfeeding as well. Remember the medications you receive during labor and delivery do pass through the placenta to the baby; they receive effects of this medication as well. Some medications are better than others and the level of sleepiness experienced by baby can depend on the medication and dose given. Medications need time to be metabolized by your baby just like they do for you. Yes, this can be a stressful time. I suggest skin-to-skin as much as possible, the less stressful the environment is for your baby the better. If your baby has not had a good feeding at the breast within the first 12 hours, consider pumping your breasts and feed this milk to your baby.

Sometimes thinking outside the box can help turn around your situation. I have seen many positive results from alternative therapies and you may need to consider one of the following options. Some health care providers will perform Cranio-Sacral Therapy (CST) on newborns. CST is an alternative therapy used by occupational therapists, physiotherapists, massage therapists and chiropractors. CST provides gentle palpation of the cranium or skull that detects rhythmic movements of the cranial bones. Selective and gentle pressure is used to manipulate the cranial bones to achieve results. This is different from acupressure. Acupressure is defined as a broad range of medicine practices sharing a common concept mainly concerned with the identification of functional beings such as digestion, breathing and eating. Again, gentle pressure is used to achieve results. Some find Physical Therapy helpful as well. The primary focus of physical therapy is on repair and promotion of mobility, function and quality of movements. If you feel your child has some level of limited mobility and needs help to perform the activity of successful breastfeeding, seeing a Physical Therapist may be helpful.

Since most deliveries are uneventful, you may never need to put this information into practice, however it is always better to be prepared for the unexpected. Now you have an idea of what you might be able to do if you are presented with any of these situations.

Another question that is frequently asked is "How much nipple pain is normal?" Since sore nipples are one of the most common complaints in breastfeeding, it deserves to have an entire chapter devoted to it.

Chapter 19: How much nipple pain is normal?

Your nipples are a very sensitive part of your body. It may take a little time for this delicate tissue to adapt to this new experience. This tenderness should ease up within a short period of time. Let's go one step further and define how much nipple discomfort is to be expected. What you should not do is to just 'grin and bear it' or listen to others who might tell you what you're experiencing is 'normal'. Many women who have come for assistance with sore nipples should have come in much sooner. So let's talk nipples...

I have discussed nipple pain briefly, but let's explore deeper into the possibilities for why you have nipple pain or tenderness. Here are some possible reasons and what can you do to help correct the situation.

Check your latch with every feeding, especially those middle of the night feedings when you might not be as alert and focused. Sometimes just one or two poor latches can cause damage that can affect future feedings. Ask yourself those three questions discussed previously in this book: what is your nipple pain level, are you experiencing productive nursing and what is your nipple shape. Be sure the answer to all these questions is 'yes'. You will need to take charge of this assessment because no one else can feel what you are feeling. It may look like a good latch to the observer, but your pain level tells a different story. If you can't get a comfortable latch by yourself or with minimal assistance, seek help from a knowledgeable health care provider or lactation consultant.

Using a position(s) that's comfortable is another part to preventing sore nipples. Practice different positions until you find something that works for both you and your baby. Some moms find a good position right away while others find it takes a few attempts. Some moms feel alternating between two positions helpful, as it distributes pressure on different parts of the nipple.

Another reason for sore nipples might be a tight frenulum. Parents and even health care providers might miss this when looking for reasons for sore nipples. The frenulum is the thin membrane that anchors the tongue to the floor of the mouth. If this attachment is too close to the tip of their tongue, it will restrict movement needed for successful and pain-free breastfeeding. The medical term for this limited tongue movement is Ankyloglossia, or tongue-tied. If this is interfering with breastfeeding, it is best to have this assessed by your health care provider when your baby is a newborn. They will determine if it is necessary to have this membrane clipped, freeing up movement of the tongue.

Many health care providers do not perform this clipping, and some parents find it easiest to see and ENT (Ear, Nose, Throat) Doctor for this to be done. The ENT doctors are very familiar with this procedure and have most likely performed this hundreds of times. It is a very simple procedure, done right in the office, if it is done when baby is a newborn. Some parents will wait and discover this tongue-tie has impacted their child's speech and has to be clipped when they're a toddler. A good ENT Doctor will be able to advise you on what is best for your baby.

Sometimes women have flatter nipples and this can potentially make it more difficult for baby to latch on. This will be largely dependent upon the baby. Lactation consultants often see babies who have difficulty breastfeeding, even though mother's nipples perfectly shaped; while other babies would nurse on something as flat as the wall if given the opportunity. Flatter nipples are not necessarily a red flag for difficulty. Nipples, in general will pull out more with nursing your baby or with pumping. This is especially true if this is your first time breastfeeding. The nipples you had when you started nursing will likely be more everted or prominent throughout your breastfeeding experience. Some women will manually roll or pull out their nipples before latching baby, while others will briefly use a breast pump before latching. Both ways to evert nipples have proven helpful. Using the positions described in the previous chapter will guide you as well.

Throughout your pregnancy your body has gone through tremendous changes. One of these changes or side effects of pregnancy is retaining fluid or swelling. When your body is retaining fluid it does so all over your body, even in your nipples. If you had a medication called Pitocin to speed along or induce your labor, you may notice this swelling or retaining of fluids is worse than before you delivered. Swelling is a possible side effect of Pitocin and as mentioned, the swelling will go everywhere in your body. Women have said, "These are not the nipples I had before I delivered!" I've seen it over and over again. The good news is that it's fairly temporary. You will soon see your old familiar nipples again.

Healing sore nipples can be done in several ways. Remember you have to be sure baby is latching correctly or you will not heal no matter how hard you try. Baby will just keep injuring you if the problems are not solved. Here are some good, inexpensive healing products:

Nipple Cream by Motherlove - This provides good healing and is ingestible, organic and safe for your baby

Coconut Oil - Provides natural healing and fairly available

Nipple Cream by Fairhaven Health - Again a good healing ointment that is organic and safe for baby

Hydrogel dressings - a gel pad that is soothing to sore nipples. The pads are worn all times unless you are nursing, pumping or showering. Each pad lasts 24-48 hours. When they are not in use, it's best to put them in a plastic baggie and put them in the refrigerator to prolong their use.

You will likely find any of these solutions helpful. I would recommend products with ingredients that are organic and stay away from ointments that are thick and sticky to the touch. These ointments frequently do not promote healing, as they do not allow enough air to get to the nipple.

The one thing that can't be stressed enough: ask for help! You do not need to go through this alone and anyone would suggest you don't. Generally there is help at a hospital, clinic, support group or independent lactation consultant. Don't wait too long before seeking advice or going in to see someone. Most women who come in for help state, after the visit, "I wish I had come to see you sooner."

Nipple soreness is one of the most common reasons new mothers quit breastfeeding during the first 1-2 weeks. Remember soreness is almost always a short-term problem. Sore nipples are a sign of issues that need to be addressed. It's important to note there are many solutions; so don't give up. You have to define the problem and trouble-shoot through some possible solutions. Many times sore nipples can resolve as quickly as they develop.

Another question almost every mother asks is "How do I know I have enough milk for my baby?" This question knows no generational, cultural or age boundaries. Nearly every mother has this concern. So let's cover this topic next.

Chapter 20: How do I know I have enough milk for my baby?

Every health care provider has heard this expressed many times and in many different ways: "No milk, no milk," says the non-English speaking Hispanic mother as she points to her breasts. "He's not even getting anything," says the teen mother as she finishes texting her girlfriend. "I don't have enough milk for her," states the first time mother with a tear in her eye. Most parents need reassuring, but I would like to offer you something more, the facts about breast milk and milk production. This will give you the information you need to help make your own accurate evaluation. I think this information will help you sleep at night.

Back when you were about 20- 24 weeks pregnant your body was busy producing colostrum. Colostrum is the first milk your breasts produce and the first few meals your baby will have. Many refer to colostrum as 'liquid gold' as it is golden in color and rich in protein, immunoglobulins and antibodies. There is nothing quite like it and it's exactly what your baby needs in the exact amount. Not only do the antibodies help protect your baby as they enter a world of bacteria and viruses, it also has a laxative effect that helps them to pass their first stools. Meconium is the baby's first few stools and can be difficult to pass, as it's black, thick and tarry. Your colostrum makes passing this stool much easier. You can see it is the perfect first food.

Another wonderful fact about your newborn is they are born with an abundant amount of brown fat. Brown fat is fat tissue with the primary function to generate body heat in newborns, as they do not have the ability to shiver. The brown fat makes up about 5% of their body mass and is located along the upper half of their spine and their back. Brown fat provides a safety net as they transition to maintaining their own body temperature.

Another interesting fact about your baby is their stomach size. The size is very small for the first 24 hours and gradually increases throughout the next few weeks. Their stomach size during the first 24 hours is 5-7 ccs. To help put this in perspective, a regular one-ounce shot glass is 30 ccs. So your baby's stomach size for the first 24 hours of life is approximately 1/6th of a shot glass. That is not very big. By day three their stomach size has grown to about 22-27 ccs; much closer to one ounce. This will help you realize that baby does not hold much food in their stomach, so the amount of milk your make in the early days is just enough for them.

When you are breastfeeding your baby you will never know an exact amount they are getting at each feeding. I suggest you let go of wanting to know the amounts and start looking for other signs breastfeeding is going well. All babies lose weight for the first 2-3 days after birth, as mentioned earlier. Frequent weight checks will be part of the discharge planning until you know baby is gaining weight at a rate of about 5-7 ounces per week. Keep track of all feedings, wet and dirty diapers until you are feeling confident and have reassuring signs that breastfeeding is going well.

Another sign that you have enough milk is to look at the color of your baby's dirty diapers. It's good to know the number of dirty diapers every 24 hours, but the color can be very telling as well. As mentioned previously, your baby's first few dirty diapers will be black and tarry. They will change to a dark brown, to a dark greenish color and then to a mustard color. Your baby should have this mustard color, seedy appearing stool by the time they are five days of age. If your baby is five days old and still having dark brown dirty diapers, you should make an appointment with your health care provider or lactation consultant to assess your situation. I can't stress enough, it's best to get help sooner rather than later.

Lastly, look for other signs Baby is doing well. Do they appear full after their feeding? They should be sleeping or be in a content alert phase after feedings. Do your breasts feel less full when baby is done nursing? Do you hear your baby swallowing when they are nursing? Is baby productively nursing or just "hanging out"? Are they content between feedings for 1 1/2 -3 hours? Are you getting at least 8 feedings every 24 hours? Being able to answer 'yes' to these questions will help you feel more confident.

There are many different signs to look for when assessing your baby's nutrition. Find a health care provider you trust and that shares your same values regarding breastfeeding. They will be a wonderful resource for you for many years to come. Sometimes babies do need extra feedings and calories. Let's take a look at some reasons to supplement a baby and appropriate amounts to supplement that won't sabotage your breastfeeding efforts.

Chapter 21: What if my baby needs to be supplemented?

With all that's been talked about throughout this book, it's easy to see why some babies struggle when making all the necessary transitions into this world. It's a tall order being born. For the most part, nearly all these situations are temporary. As health care providers, we all must be mindful to keep these babies as healthy as possible, this becomes top priority. Sometimes keeping babies healthy may involve providing a supplemental or additional feeding. This does not mean you have to abandon breastfeeding! In fact, it's extremely important to keep breastfeeding going throughout this period.

If you asked 100 lactation consultants what's the number one action that sabotages breastfeeding more than any other; 99 of them would say inappropriate supplementing. Now we do understand that providing additional nutrition and calories are needed in certain situations. We have seen supplementing become an essential intervention in the health and wellness of many babies. What I'm talking about here is inappropriate supplementing for non-medical reasons.

One reason may be a mom wanting to sleep all night and have her baby bottle feed in the nursery. Although this may seem tempting when you are tired, this is the time to get to know your baby and learn their cues for a feeding. A mother called me frantically after her first night home from the hospital. She thought something was wrong with her baby because he "ate every two hours". When asked what her nighttime feedings were like while she was in the hospital for four days after her cesarean birth, she simply stated, "I don't know. I slept for 8 hours every night. The nurses said I should get my sleep while I could." Needless to say no good came from this advice. Not only did the mother have a delay in milk production due to a lack of stimulation and receptor growth, she also wasn't familiar with her babies' normal pattern of nighttime feedings. She was amazed at his feeding frequency and her lack of production. An aggressive feeding and stimulation plan began with this mother. She began to frequently nurse her baby, pump after nursing to help make up for the deficit, and supplement her breastfeeding. This feeding plan lasted for five days before her supply caught up with the baby's demand. So you can see how much more work was necessary because of this poor advice.

There are medical reasons your baby may need a supplement. Some of these reasons might be:

- Low blood sugar
- Weight loss at or approaching 10%
- No latch in the first 24 hours
- Jaundice
- Mom not available

If your baby may need a supplement, it's still very important to supplement an appropriate amount and use an appropriate method for supplementing. We will talk in depth about amounts and methods later, but here are some general guidelines:

- Less than 24 hours of age   5-10 cc's
- 24-48 hours of age   10-20 cc's
- 48-72 hours of age   20-30 cc's
- Over 72 hours of age   Ad lib

While your baby may need to be supplemented for one or more of the reasons stated above, breastfeeding can and should be preserved. This situation is usually quite temporary and not life threatening to your baby. It may mean a little more work while you are going through the process, but the results are worth it. Meeting your breastfeeding goal will be something to be proud of and something that will empower you. Having the feeling of "I did it!" is something you will carry with you for a long time.

There are many features to breastfeeding, the more you know and are prepared for, and the more success you will have. I hope this book will assist and guide you to lay a strong foundation to help you meet your breastfeeding goals. Don't doubt yourself as a mother. Remember no one knows your baby better than you do. Trust yourself and enjoy your new adventure. It's like no other you've ever been on before!

Chapter 22: What should I do when my breasts are engorged?

The engorgement process can be rather tricky. It can vary in degrees from mild to severe, happen with some mothers and not others, and it can happen quickly or take its time. Like many Lactation Consultants, I have seen all aspects of engorgement.

So what is engorgement after all? Engorgement is defined as swelling and expanding of the breast tissue caused by production of breast milk. Or, more simply put, increased pressure due to milk coming in. Some women feel slightly firm while others say that their breasts feel hard as rocks. Some mothers describe their breasts as slightly tender while others will actually have painful breasts. There can be a difference in how quick or forceful your milk will let down for your baby. Typically, more engorgement in the breast will slow the flow of milk. One challenge of engorgement involves the nipple. As the breast fills and swells, nipples respond by becoming flatter. This may make it more difficult for baby to latch on. Some breasts even take on the appearance of a balloon full of water, ready to burst. Others have stated their breasts have taken on the rounder more firm appearance, much like the appearance of a knee. When Baby tries to latch on to that firm breast, one can see why they have trouble or become frustrated. Have no fear; here are some solutions you will find helpful.

From the beginning of your breastfeeding, it is best to have frequent feedings. Even if these feedings are brief, the relief a short feeding gives you may be all that is necessary to prevent engorgement. Remember this is the number one way to control and even prevent engorgement. Your breasts are meant to produce and distribute milk; they are not meant to store milk. When your breasts are asked to perform this storage function, due to delayed or infrequent feedings, they may begin to slow production. This causes swelling and tenderness. Frequent emptying is your best defense against engorgement.

Another intervention is to use cool packs. When swelling happens anywhere on your body, essentially you treat it in the same manner. Whether it is a sprained ankle, jammed finger or a twisted knee; the common intervention is to cool the area. Cool packs or ice packs will be very helpful in decreasing the swelling and tenderness when you are treating engorgement. Using cold to your area of trauma also acts as a means of pain control. Use cool packs as much or as little, providing you are getting relief.

Treating engorgement with warmth may be helpful, but please be aware of this caution. Using warmth for more than a few minutes may actually cause more swelling. The primary reason you would use warmth is to help dilate the milk sinuses and milk ducts just before you are going to breastfeed or pump. This dilating allows more milk flow. This will enable better emptying of the breast, which will relieve the pressure and make your more comfortable. However, be sure to use warmth for only around 3-5 minutes and only immediately before nursing.

Another measure you can take is to do some gentle, light massage in circular motions around your breast just before nursing or pumping. This light massage prepares the breast for better emptying. Be sure the massage remains gentle, as deep tissue massage may increase the swelling.

Lastly, some women find drinking mangosteen juice helps to decrease the swelling inside your breast. Usually drinking one to three ounces, three times per day makes a noticeable difference. The taste is palatable and might be only needed for a few days.

The important piece to take away from this chapter is how to prevent engorgement from happening in the first place. You can avoid all those potential issues and interventions to help deal with engorgement if you nurse frequently. After all, eating frequently is the normal pattern of a newborn; there's no getting around that, since their stomach size is so small and their growth rate is so rapid. Remember also you always have a resource in your lactation consultant. Having an observer watch the baby nurse can give insight to how baby is emptying the breast. Returning to the basics learned in the first days of breastfeeding can prevent many problems.

Another issue that could come up is the problem of slow weight gain for your baby. When this happens, it can be a fearful time for everyone, especially the parents. The next chapter will tell you step by step how to turn your worrisome situation around.

Chapter 23: What should I do if my baby isn't gaining weight?

As mentioned throughout this entire series, you need frequent weight checks for your baby until you know everything is going well. Some old school doctors will still say to come in for a two-week check up. That may be ok for a few babies, however it's important to know that there can be weight gain problems long before your baby is two weeks old. The American Academy of Pediatrics (AAP) recommends newborns have a weight check 2-4 days after being discharged from a hospital or birthing center. If you had a home birth, you may also need frequent weight checks until baby is gaining well. Most midwives who provide home deliveries will provide this service as well. There are several reasons for a baby to have little or no weight gain in those first weeks. Let's look at a few of them.

One of the more common reasons baby isn't gaining weight is ineffective breastfeeding. This happens when baby is on the breast, but not nursing productively. Remember your baby should exhibit large jaw movements, active motion at their temple muscles, and you should hear swallowing. The red flags for ineffective breastfeeding are; not feeling some tugging or pulling at the breast, not feeling emptied after the feeding or not seeing the baby's jaw activity as described. Slow weight gain upon having baby's weight checked, or seeing a decreased number of wet and dirty diapers; less than 5-6 wet and 3-4 dirty, may also lead you to this conclusion.

When there is ineffective breastfeeding, this usually leads to a delay in milk coming in or low milk production. Poor stimulation to the breasts can cause the hormone prolactin to diminish enough to reduce your supply.

Infrequent feedings can also lead to baby not gaining enough weight. Any baby, even formula fed babies, will need eight feedings every 24 hours. Be sure your baby has at least this many feedings. It's important to keep track of all feedings. It's easy to lose track of time and forget when one feeding ended and the other began, so write them down. If your baby is getting fewer than eight feedings a day, or spaced more than three hours apart, this is not enough. You may need to wake your baby for some of their feedings, especially during the daytime. This is common while they are still trying to regain their birth weight. A perfect waking technique is skin-to-skin!

Another possible reason why your baby may not be gaining weight might be that they are tongue-tied. This topic was discussed earlier, under sore nipples. To recap briefly, a baby is tongue tied when their frenulum, the membrane under the tongue, is too close to the end of their tongue, causing limited movement. Without proper full range of motion of the tongue, baby can't stimulate the breasts effectively. This leads to decreased stimulation, lower milk supply and inappropriate weight gain. It's easy to see how one event affects the other and how it can all snowball in the wrong direction.

If you find your baby in a situation of slow weight gain, what options do you have? You have to preserve the breastfeeding process, while putting some 'safety nets' in place. When you have a one or more of the issues described above, most likely you will need a three step-feeding plan.

#1 - How to preserve breastfeeding. Even if you're breastfeeding for only a few minutes at each feeding, your baby is practicing while continuing to make the connection between you and nourishment. Continue to offer the breast first. Let baby nurse as long as they are productively nursing, as identified previously. When your baby isn't gaining weight properly, they are likely very sleepy. This may mean baby is only nursing for a few minutes, perhaps only 2-3. When your baby becomes sleepy and is no longer nursing well, end the feeding. The biggest mistake parents make when working with a sleepy baby is to let baby stay at the breast only "attempting" for too long a time. This sleepy and ineffective comfort sucking and is not recommended for two reasons:

- When baby 'comfort sucks', they are using more calories than they are receiving. This will potentially drive their weight down even further.
- After these short attempts at breastfeeding, a good double electric pump will stimulate you better and drive your hormones up higher than your baby will. This means pumping will build up your milk supply sooner than your sleepy baby.

In other words, you determine when to end the feeding at the breast based on your baby's behavior, not based on the clock. Some mothers will give their baby a grade for how well they are breastfeeding: A, B, C or D. If your baby is nursing productively, giving effort and having more sucking than pausing, you would grade them an A or B. If they were only comfort sucking, falling asleep and pausing more than they are sucking, you would grade them a C or D. End the feeding when they are a C or D, as they don't have enough energy for the feeding. Now is where the safety nets come into play.

#2 - The second step is supplementing your baby; this is your first safety net. When you supplement or give them additional milk after you have nursed, you are providing the extra calories they need to begin gaining weight. Use any milk you have pumped or previously pumped for their supplement. If you don't have any of your previously pumped breast milk, you will need to use donor milk, expressed milk from a trusted friend or lastly infant formula. If you get started on a feeding plan right when you discover the problem, it is likely you will pump enough for your little one.

#3 - Provide stimulation to your breasts that you are not getting from your baby. That means using a breast pump. This is your second safety net. Remember, supply is based on demand; the more demand put on the breast, the more you will supply. The pump will now take over where your baby left off. Pumping will bring your hormone level up to where it's needed for effective milk production. If possible, try to pump right after you have ended the feeding with your baby. Your hormones are primed and ready for more stimulation. Most women find the best stimulation is with a double electric breast pump. Using rental or hospital grade pumps will provide the best stimulation. Pump both breasts for 10-15 minutes after nursing. Save any milk you may collect to use when you supplement your baby.

I would like to dig deeper into the entire supplementing process. Supplementing does not mean you abandon breastfeeding. I strongly encourage you not to do this. It is simply a short-term solution to get your baby to gain weight. It may also be a temporary treatment for newborn jaundice. There are two important aspects of supplementing that need to be addressed: how much milk to give and how to give it.

Supplementing age appropriate amounts is very important. Your baby's stomach size is much smaller than you may realize. Below are guidelines to follow for appropriate supplement amounts. These are designed for your baby's age and stomach size, and are recommended by the American Academy of Pediatrics and also followed by the Academy of Breastfeeding Medicine.

- Less than 24 hours of age   5-10 cc's
- 24-48 hours of age   10-20 cc's
- 48-72 hours of age   20-30 cc's
- Over 72 hours of age   Ad lib

Using these amounts will allow your baby to gain, without being overfed. When babies are overfed they tend to shut down, get gassy, bloated and not be ready for their next feeding. These amounts given after your baby has been to the breast, this will likely eliminate those overfed side effects. Whenever your baby is on a feeding plan, frequent weight checks will be essential. Continue to keep track of all feedings, wet and dirty diapers until your baby has established a good weight-gaining pattern.

The method you chose to supplement your baby may have potential detriment to the breastfeeding process. I suggest cup, dropper/finger feeding or, spoon or over using a bottle. Many babies have difficulty going back and forth between breasts to bottle. They can get confused by the firmness or the fast flow a bottle nipple often delivers. Either too slow or too fast could be problematic if using a poorly designed nipple. Remember you don't want to sabotage breastfeeding. Your choice to use the following methods instead of a bottle will preserve breastfeeding:

- Cup feeding is done by using a small, soft, pliable cup like a Foley cup or medicine cup and Baby actually laps up or drinks. It works well if they are wrapped up a bit. Baby is in more of a sitting position as you bring a small amount of supplement to the tip of their lips. Baby opens and begins lapping it up. This is favorable, as nothing foreign is entering their mouth to provide an opportunity for potential confusion.
- Dropper feeding is done by using a small, soft, pliable syringe or medicine dropper. It is best when Baby is sucking on a finger so they begin to make the connection between sucking and getting nutrition. When Baby sucks, guide the tip of the dropper along side of your finger. Baby continues to suck while you are slowly dropping the supplement. Refill the dropper as needed.
- Sometimes using a spoon can be effective. Often this is done when the supplement amount is small as in early feedings of colostrum. If baby is given too much at one time, they may cough or choke, or not know how to handle the amount. This can be alarming for both Baby and the parents.
- If using a bottle, be sure it has a slow flow nipple and has a larger base to the nipple. Utilizing these features may help Baby to go back and forth from bottle to breast more easily.

A feeding plan for a slow weight-gaining baby may look daunting at first, however following it one feeding at a time then one day at a time will encourage you, and you will see results. Your baby will have more alert time, more wet and dirty diapers and he will become more interested in each breastfeeding session. Feeding plans are generally used on a short-term basis, around 1-5 days until you achieve your final results.

Since breast milk production is such an individual matter, milk supply can vary greatly among nursing women. While some may struggle to make milk, others are drowning their baby with a more-than-ample milk supply. This over supply can create just as many problems. Let's take a look at what to do if this is your problem.

Chapter 24: What should I do if I have too much milk?

Producing too much milk may seem like a wonderful problem to have, but the truth is it may cause an entirely different set of problems. A mother may know she is struggling for some reason, but just doesn't realize what it might be. Most people have heard stories from neighbors, coworkers and friends about low milk supply that having too much milk isn't even on their radar. There are many women who do have this issue, enough women for us to have an entire chapter dedicated to the subject.

Sometimes called hyperlactation, a mother simply produces more milk than her baby needs. Some mothers state this is actually stressful and we can understand why. When let down occurs it is immediately followed by a rush of milk. This rush of milk can be uncomfortable as the floodgates open wide and baby often times has trouble keeping up with the intense flow. Some babies gulp or swig, while others choke, sputter or even get upset and pull away from the breast. If this is happening to you, don't take it personally, your baby is just trying to survive and adapt. Here are some signs you may be dealing with hyperlactation and some actions you can take to help deal with this issue.

If your baby frequently chokes, coughs, or struggles at the breast, they may compensate for a rapid flow by biting or clamping down on the breast. This is the same principle as clamping off a garden hose that may be flowing too quickly. Those babies are smart! When they are hungry and want to eat, they realize the need to control the rapid flow. Their solution is to pinch off the tip of the nipple by pressing their tongue against the roof of their mouth. This allows them time to swallow and breathe before taking in another mouthful. If this is happening, you will find your nipple coming out pinched or creased and sometimes even white in color.

Crying, restlessness during feeding, and irritability are other behaviors your baby might have due to the over supply of milk. Some babies may tense up and become stiff during feeding. Common behaviors of an overfed baby can be spitting up, gassiness, large burps and green, watery explosive bowel movements. This is due to the large amount of air they are taking in while they are gulping during feedings. When stool moves rapidly through the baby's digestive system, water does not get reabsorbed causing the watery consistency. In addition, the stool becomes green as it picks up bile and bacteria during the same rapid digestion. The usual stool of a breast fed baby will look like cottage cheese mixed with mustard; yellow in color and lose but not watery.

Another aspect mothers may deal with related to hyperlactation is milk spraying when baby comes off of the breast. Some mothers may spray milk before their baby even nurses. Simply taking pressure off the breast by lowering your bra flap may cause spraying to occur. You may devote an entire load of laundry to burp cloths each day.

You may also notice baby only needs to feed on one side, or nurses for short periods on each breast. Your baby is quickly getting satisfied because your milk is so plentiful; so don't worry about the clock. Your breasts might even feel full a good deal of the time. Women either get accustomed to this and their breasts adapt, or they pump occasionally after feedings. Although pumping may help it may also increase your milk supply even further. Instead, here are some more productive ways to help deal with an over abundant milk supply.

One strategy is to nurse your baby using only one side for a designated period of time; let's say 2 hours. Use only one breast per feeding during this time period. When your baby needs to return to the breast and it's under the 2 hours since they fed, use the same breast. If you feel too full on the other breast, you can pump or hand express your breast briefly, but only for comfort. Comfort might mean you need to pump for 2-3 minutes. This pattern will tend to decrease your milk until you no longer feel the need to pump that second breast. Be sure you are pumping only until you feel the pressure is less, a long period of pumping will send a signal to your breasts to continue the same production, or possibly to produce even more. Remember when your breasts are fuller, it sends a message to your brain that says to slow down production. This pattern will help down-regulate your supply safely. You should notice a difference in around four to seven days.

If you haven't gotten the relief you are looking for, try this strategy. Allow your baby to nurse on one side for only 1-3 minutes, switch sides and allow them to complete their feeding on the second side. This will eliminate any pumping you may find you needed in the first strategy. It's important to let baby nurse for a longer period of time on the second breast. This will allow your baby to receive the hind milk, which is the higher fat milk.

If neither of these measures are working for you, consult your local lactation consultant to help you manage your over supply. Below are some suggestions for herbals or medications that may decrease your supply. However, I don't recommend trying them without consulting a lactation consultant. If used without guidance these medications could swing you into a low milk supply, which can be even harder to manage and reverse. You don't want to lose too much milk at once, so these items should be used carefully with professional supervision.

- Low dose birth control pill containing estrogen and progesterone for 3-5 days
- Sage, either in tea or tincture form
- Pseudo-ephedrine, such as Sudafed
- Antihistamine such as Benadryl

Again, I would not recommend using any of the above without supervision as everyone reacts differently, everyone's supply is different and you don't want to lose too much milk at once.

If you don't have an over supply issue but your baby still struggles during nursing, you may still be affected by overactive let down. Overactive let down is forceful ejection of milk from the breast. In some women, it only occurs during the first one to two let downs, but occasionally they may experience strong let downs throughout the feeding. Some symptoms are the same as discussed before; your baby might gulp, choke and be gassy. They may even pinch off your nipple to help control the flow. The difference between this and producing too much milk is that babies usually go to both breasts with each feeding and your breasts feel less full when baby is done. In other words, supply is matching the demands of your baby.

The most effective action you can take for overactive let down is to modify both of your positions. Place your baby in a more upright position allowing them to have better control of the flow. The football hold is usually very helpful, allowing the baby to have their head as high, or higher than your breast. While you are using the football hold, you should also recline or lean back. Use an actual recliner or place multiple pillows at the head of your bed allowing you to lean back. This will require your milk to "travel uphill" and naturally slow down the flow. Another effective hold is a modified cross cradle. Hold your baby so their bottom is low and their head is higher than the breast. You should adjust your position so you are more reclined. This position will naturally slow down the flow, allowing baby to have better control. If your baby chokes or coughs, unlatch them and allow your excess milk to spray into a towel or burp cloth. When the milk stops flowing, re-latch baby.

Some mothers will try to pinch off the flow by using a scissors hold on the areola (the dark area around the nipple). By placing the nipple between two fingers, you will decrease the flow, depending on how hard and long you press the areola. Use this method with caution, as you don't want to press too hard or too long as this may cause pain or plugged milk ducts.

There are plenty of moms out there who can relate to this chapter for one or more reasons. Most of them are saying, "So that's what the problem was!" I'm glad I could help put the pieces together for you and provide some solutions. Please don't forget about the option of donating some of your abundant milk supply to help other babies who desperately need your amazing gift of life. Donating your breast milk is easy to do and won't have any cost to you. Visit www.hmbana.org and take the first step in making this life changing decision.

What if you don't fit into either of the 'too little or too much' milk categories? What if you are Goldilocks and your supply is just right but you are still having some issues with breastfeeding? In the next chapter I will cover some other challenges you might be facing to help you think beyond a supply problem.

Chapter 25: I think I have plugged ducts or mastitis or thrush. What should I do?

Concerns and worries may come up throughout your entire breastfeeding experience. They might not show up for several weeks or months, or you may be a mother who just sails through breastfeeding with no issues. Congratulations, you are one of the fortunate nursing mothers.

But also, life happens! Other children get sick or you get sick, so stress and fatigue are very real. Women are returning to work and the pressure or worry from that life change may lead you to uncharted territory. Let's talk about some of the problems that can occur from just being overly tired or stressed, and what you can do to help reverse your situation entirely.

A plugged milk duct occurs when the milk duct is not draining well. This lack of draining leads to milk stasis, and that leads to plugging of the milk duct. Some symptoms include:

- Localized inflammation and swelling
- Warm to touch
- Tenderness in the affected area
- Lumpy or knotty area

If draining does not occur, it can lead to more swelling with more pressure and potentially mastitis, which is an infection within the breast. This may cause a larger area of the breast to become tender or painful. The good news is that most women will never have a plugged milk duct. Others, however, may have reoccurring episodes. If you do find you have a plugged milk duct, it's best to attempt to unplug the area as soon as possible. The best ways to help unplug a milk duct are as follows:

- Use cool packs or ice packs to the area. This will provide comfort while decreasing the swelling around the affected area.
- Start baby on the affected breast first until the plug has resolved. Babies typically have a stronger suck and a more aggressive pattern on the first side. When they are hungry and thirsty strong sucking will likely move the milk through the duct.
- Changing positions for breastfeeding may also help. This will change the "pressure points" and will allow different areas of the breast to be accessed.
- Light massage before and during the nursing session may help to move the milk through also. Be sure not to do any deep tissue massage, as this may cause more swelling.
- Using warmth briefly, under 5 minutes, before pumping and/or breastfeeding may help as well. The warmth helps to dilate the milk duct, allowing the milk to pass. Using it longer than 5 minutes may cause more swelling.
- Mangosteen is a tropical fruit native to Southeast Asia and is marketed as a supplement, both as juice and in capsule form. A number of studies suggest mangosteen has significant anti-inflammatory effects, which will help decrease the swelling.

If you are a mother who has recurrent plugged milk ducts, you may find Soy Lecithin to be helpful. Lecithin is a common food additive and is found naturally in many foods. There are no known contraindications for using Lecithin. Some women need to take two to three 1200 mg capsules per day to help get the plugged ducts under control. Once you are symptom-free for two weeks, you can decrease by one capsule each week. You may find taking one capsule per day as a maintenance dose may prevent those plugged ducts from reoccurring.

Mastitis is another issue some mothers may experience, and wish they hadn't. Mastitis is inflammation leading to an infection within the breast.

Mastitis can occur because the baby is not latched properly, has infrequent feedings and has difficulty removing the milk from the breast. As mentioned, mastitis can be the result of a prolonged plugged milk duct. Stress and fatigue play a part in this as well. Mastitis usually affects only one breast and symptoms can develop quickly so don't hesitate to seek help. Typical symptoms include:

- Breast tenderness and swelling
- Affected area is warm to touch and lumpy
- Skin redness, often in a wedge-shaped pattern
- Pain or burning sensation at the site
- Fever of 101 or greater
- Flu-like symptoms of aches, chills and fatigue

If you are experiencing these symptoms, especially the last three, you should contact your health care provider. It is likely you will need a course of antibiotics to get this resolved. A high fever and flu-like symptoms are the biggest difference between plugged ducts, and mastitis. Remember, you do not have an infection in your milk, only in the tissue of your breast. You should continue breastfeeding your baby during your treatment. The antibiotics used are safe for your baby.

Along with plugged ducts and mastitis, some women deal with thrush. Thrush, also known as Candidiasis is a fungal infection. It is commonly referred to as a yeast infection. Candida is a fungus that occurs naturally in the mucous membranes and on skin. The use of antibiotics increases the growth of yeast by killing off the good bacteria that helps keep yeast from multiplying too rapidly. Some symptoms in baby:

- Creamy white spots or patches inside the mouth/tongue
- Spots may look shiny with reddened areas around them
- Fussy or gassy behavior
- Signs of discomfort when sucking
- Diaper rash that is slightly raised, red or shiny
- Actively pulling away from the breast

Mother will experience:
- Burning pains on the nipple or deep into the breast
- Burning that starts in the nipple and shoots back toward the spine
- Pain may or may not occur during breastfeeding
- Tender irritated nipples that are sensitive to touching or rubbing
- Areola is shiny with small raised bumps that could be itchy or puffy
- A decrease in milk supply
- Sore nipples after a period of pain-free nursing
- Pain that tends to be worse at night

Sometimes the nipples don't look as bad as they feel. Don't underestimate the severity of this, as yeast is hard to eliminate. Seek assistance soon. When treating yeast, one of the most important things to remember is to always treat both mom and baby. Sometimes the health care provider will treat just one of the pair. This never solves the problem as you continue to transfer the infection to each other. In this case, you and baby are one unit and need to both be treated for the same length of time. You may need to contact your pediatrician and your obstetrician to obtain prescriptions from both. If you have a family practice physician or a midwife, they may prescribe for both of you.

The treatment options for Thrush are as follows:
- Baby needs Nystatin oral suspension. The instructions may say to apply 4 times per day after feedings. It's actually more effective to give 1/2 applications 8 times per day to neutralize their mouth after all feedings.
- Gentian Violet can be an effective treatment for baby, but is messy and stains.
- Mother needs a topical anti-fungal such as Miconazole to apply after each nursing session.
- Motherlove Diaper Rash and Thrush cream may be used topically for both mom and baby. I have seen good results with this. Myrrh is the herbal anti-fungal ingredient and the other herbals help with

symptoms of itching, burning and irritation. Be sure to use a separate jar for mom and baby.

- Use pumped milk from a previous time, while you are being treated. While you are both being treated, use pumped milk from the time period you were infected. Using this milk later on may cause the yeast to return.
- Boil all bottles, nipples, oral toys and pacifiers for 5 minutes to kill the fungus.
- Boil breast pump parts for 5 minutes.
- Wash all bras and nursing pads in hot water.

If you are not receiving relief and the symptoms are not clearing within 48-72 hours, you need an oral anti-fungal. Fluconazole, also called Diflucan or Trican may need to be prescribed. Dr. Jack Newman, a well-known physician specializing in lactation, suggests using a 400 mg loading dose followed by 100 mg twice a day until you are pain free for one week. This treatment becomes more effective if you also add probiotics to your diet. Thrush can be tricky to diagnose and treat, so don't hesitate to seek help from your health professional or a qualified Lactation Consultant.

Most of you will not be bothered by any of the challenges cited. However, if you are one of those breastfeeding moms dealing with any of these issues, you will be glad to have these answers at your fingertips.

Some problems can be solved by using a nipple shield. You might be one who could benefit from this simple little tool.

Chapter 26: Would using a nipple shield help my situation?

A nipple shield is a thin nipple-shaped covering that is worn over your nipple during breastfeeding. It has holes in the end to allow milk to be transferred to baby. Some of you may gasp at the thought of using a nipple shield. You heard nipple shields are bad for breastfeeding, they decrease your milk supply and baby becomes dependent on them right? Nipple shields have a controversial history, no doubt about that. This controversy came about mainly because of the material the shields were made from. Nipple shields go back as far as the 17th century when they were first made of pewter. Then they were made of a thick rubber or latex. Often times that thickness would lead to poor milk transfer because of poor stimulation of the breast. The change in thinking began when the Journal of Human Lactation (1996 fall issue), devoted their entire issue to nipple shields. Today nipple shields are made of a very thin silicone, which preserves the breastfeeding process and allows enough stimulation for a full milk supply. There is a time, place, and situation where nipple shields are the remedy. They should not be used carelessly and to potentially solve all breastfeeding issues.

There are many situations when using a nipple shield can be very beneficial. Sometimes nipple shields are needed for reasons the mother may exhibit, while others times for baby-identified reasons.

Mother reasons:
- Flatter nipples
- Edematous or swollen nipples due to epidurals and Pitocin during labor

- Sore nipples that don't improve with intervention
- Slowing an overactive let down

Baby reasons:
- High arched palate
- Shorter tongue or tongue tied
- Multiple bottles early on causing baby to be bottle impressed
- Early introduction of a pacifier
- Uncoordinated suck due to premature birth or traumatic birth

Some of you are afraid to use a nipple shield, but research has found them to be a useful tool, especially for the premature infant. It has been demonstrated that premature babies got more volume at breast using a nipple shield. It has also been found that when using the shield, baby progressed faster with their feedings, and growth, and went home sooner. In most cases, babies are weaned from the shield close to their original due date.

If you are using a nipple shield it's important to know that baby is getting enough milk and you are getting enough stimulation. These can be determined easily and quickly by keeping track of feedings, wet and dirty diapers and frequent weight checks.

Nipple shields come in three sizes: 16 mm, 20 mm and 24 mm. The 16 mm is quite small and most women will not fit comfortably into this size. The more common size is a 20 mm, followed by the 24 mm. The size is determined by measuring the diameter of your nipple across the base, in millimeters. Your size may change throughout your breastfeeding. Your nipple should not be so snug inside the shield that it becomes painful, nor should it be so loose that you have trouble keeping it in place.

Once your problems have been resolved and baby is gaining weight you can attempt to wean baby off the shield. This is best accomplished by frequent attempts without using the shield or beginning the feeding using the shield then removing it soon into the feeding. Your baby will let you know when they are ready to fly solo.

So, don't be afraid if you find you need to use a nipple shield for a while. The use of shields has advanced so much over the years and they have become a very effective device. One mom told me, "Using this nipple shield has really saved my breastfeeding relationship." Many women who need to use a shield feel this way and tell you they would do the same thing again. I'm just glad they're no longer making them of pewter! I'd like to take the next chapter to cover some of those remaining questions you might still have.

Chapter 27: I have so many more questions, where should I start?

Along with having a baby, you most likely have a multitude of questions. This is very normal and it is good that you are searching for answers. The little bundle of joy is not born with an owner's manual: although that would be nice. Here are answers to some of the more common questions moms have. These questions were chosen based on my nearly 20 years of experience as a practicing Lactation Consultant. My day is filled with answering questions from new mothers on the phone, helping moms while they are in the hospital and following their progress after discharge. I'm certain their questions will be some of your questions as well.

Providing ways to comfort your baby seems like it should come naturally. Remember your baby has a unique personality and you will likely use a trial-and-error method to discover comfort measures specific to your baby. It will get easier as you get to know your baby and their own little personality. So be patient with yourself. Once you have taken care of the immediate demands of hunger, burping and changing their diaper, you might find some of these comfort measures helpful. Remember they are comforted by your calm voice, your heartbeat and being held. They know when you are tense and frustrated, so try to remain as calm as possible.

Doing skin-to-skin with your baby is a sure-fire way to calm them down. If you recall, skin-to-skin decreases baby's stress hormones by over 60%! They hear your heartbeat, hear your voice and smell your familiar scent. It's home sweet home, the best place to be for them. Here are some other helpful hints you may find useful:

- Avoid over feeding your baby. This will cause them to feel bloated and uncomfortable. Keep track of feedings, as each feeding may run into the other and it will be easy to think they must be hungry. Feeding a baby that is not hungry will likely cause them to be fussier.
- Swaddle your baby until they calm down. However, don't have your baby sleep swaddled tightly.
- Change your environment - go outside or in the car if possible.
- Try firmly patting or rubbing their back to release a trapped burp.
- If you can't do skin-to-skin, hold them close against your chest so they can hear your heartbeat. Playing sounds that mimic the womb are especially helpful.
- Calm them by giving a massage; working head to toe usually works best. Massaging may help them to pass trapped gas.
- Rocking motions are almost always helpful. You may find a swing, stroller or wearing a Moby wrap are all helpful ways to calm your baby. Remember they were used to activity and motion while they were inside of you.
- Sounds of familiar voices, singing or calmly talking to your baby will be familiar to them and they often respond by calming down to listen to you.
- Give them a bath. The warm water is comfortable and calming and may also help relieve some trapped gas. You could give that massage after their bath to complete the event.

It's important to remember your baby isn't crying to make your life difficult or to make you feel inadequate as their parent. They are crying because there is something wrong. You may not be able to actually see what is wrong, so you will have to trouble shoot through some potential possibilities. Newborns have immature nervous systems and can be disorganized. It may appear they don't know what they want. Never forget, when in doubt, they want you! You are their world, their everything. No one else knows your baby the way that you do, so trust yourself. These times don't last forever. Be patient with your baby and with yourself, as you get to know this precious gift that has been given to you.

Babies grow at an amazing rate. Most babies will triple their birth weight by one year of age; other babies may by 9 months or sooner. Growth spurts happen to all babies and can be puzzling to parents. Just when you think you've got things figured out, it's time for another growth spurt. During a growth spurt, a baby will suddenly begin to feed more often and for longer periods of time. They may also be fussier than before. They may have changes to their sleep patterns becoming very erratic and unpredictable.

Generally, the major growth spurts occur at 2-3 weeks, 6 weeks, then again at 3 and 6 months. Particularly at these times mothers might feel they are experiencing a decrease in their milk supply. Usually these growth spurts only last a couple of days, so when in doubt, feed again. Putting your baby back to the breast will increase your milk supply to meet baby's temporary need for more calories. After this period of non-stop eating, your baby may sleep more soundly. It is believed that while sleeping, the actual growing occurs. Nearly 80% of the growth hormone is secreted during sleep. Therefore your baby needs sleep to enable their body to produce that hormone.

Many women wonder when is the best time to begin pumping. Here are some general rules in regards to pumping. It is best not to begin pumping until your milk is fully in; your baby is eating well, and is back to their birth weight. As stated previously, your hormone prolactin is high right after birth and will slowly decrease until about day 7-10 where it will then stabilize. If you are pumping while your hormone level is high along with your baby nursing, you may begin to overproduce. Having an issue of under-producing is a problem, and over producing can be just as problematic. Waiting those 7-10 days will help you produce the right amount of milk for your baby.

Sometimes it becomes necessary to pump sooner, this should be done under the supervision of a health care professional or preferably a lactation consultant to guide you. If your baby isn't gaining, your milk isn't coming in, or you have a history of breast surgery or low milk supply, earlier pumping may be necessary for your success.

If all is going well and your baby is back to their birth weight by 2 weeks of age, pumping can safely be initiated. Breast pumps were covered in depth, but overall it is best to have a double electric pump for the best stimulation. A double pump takes half the time and uses less of your energy than a manual pump. When you pump it's recommended to pump both sides at the same time for 10-15 minutes total. When pumping, you are either doing so in place of a feeding, or pumping after your baby is finished nursing. You don't want to pump before a feeding or in between feedings. If you are pumping in place of a feeding, pump as close to baby's natural feeding time as possible. If you are pumping after a feeding to help collect some extra milk, try to pump within 15-20 minutes after the feeding. Every time you breastfeed, your hormone prolactin elevates and remains elevated for 15-20 minutes. Therefore immediate pumping will help you capitalize on the high hormone level, stimulate you better, and increase your supply. If you want to build a supply of milk for your freezer without over-producing, pump 1-3 times per day after baby is done feeding. Prolactin levels have a high and low throughout a twenty-four hour period. They are highest in the early morning hours, and lowest during the late afternoon and early evening hours. Therefore, pumping after a morning feeding will give you more leftovers than pumping after an evening.

When is it right to offer a bottle so that someone else can feed the baby? Many moms have read about nipple confusion and don't want this for their baby. The most risky time for this to occur is during the first 1-2 weeks of life. Methods of supplementation were covered in depth and reasons given why you should postpone using a bottle. Waiting until breastfeeding is well established and baby is back to their birth weight before introducing a bottle will set you up for a successful transition.

Babies usually take a bottle best when expressed breast milk is in the bottle and if offered by someone other than mother. Sometimes they can even sense and smell if you're in the room. Waiting too long to offer a bottle may be an issue as well. Waiting for many months, or until just before returning to work may not prove to be very successful, as babies usually show a strong preference for breastfeeding. If you want your baby to go back and forth between breast and bottle, it is best to introduce a bottle sometime between 2-4 weeks of age. You will likely have to keep offering bottles as part of their routine, so they remember that taking bottles is ok. If you give them one bottle, then not another for 2 months, they may not remember the newly learned behavior. Keep it fresh in their minds; perhaps giving a bottle somewhat regularly, say every 1-3 days. Some babies go back and forth without difficulty, others struggle with a bottle. You don't know how your baby may respond to moving between breast and bottle, so I suggest offering the bottle feedings with some consistency.

When to wean from breastfeeding is you and your baby's decision, but it's best if this happens gradually. It is not recommended to wean all at once as this usually causes your breasts to become engorged and uncomfortable. A slow weaning process is best. When you slowly wean, you substitute a nursing session with a bottle or Sippy cup every few days. When you skip a feeding, and feel uncomfortably full, you can express just enough milk to give you relief until you breastfeed again. Alternating a breastfeeding with a bottle or cup feeding is best for you to avoid becoming too engorged. Continue to wean by dropping one feeding each week until you are finished with breastfeeding. This slow weaning process is the safest way to wean from breastfeeding and helps to avoid potential problems. The feedings just before bed or during the nighttime are usually the last to go. Many mothers feed their baby just 1-2 times per day for many months. Those two feedings could be early morning and bedtime. Keeping the feedings you and your baby like best will give comfort to both of you as you wean from breastfeeding.

There have been many issues, concerns and potential problems addressed throughout this book. My hope is that you can use this as a guide if any of these issues arise at any point throughout your breastfeeding experience. These suggestions and interventions will benefit you and your baby, along with preserving breastfeeding for as long as you both desire. Getting to know your baby through breastfeeding is one of the most satisfying life experiences.

Chapter 28: How do I know if I have a low milk supply?

It's important to remember that nearly every woman is capable of making enough milk for their baby. Also remember that babies fuss for many reasons other than hunger, so you don't jump to any conclusions based on occasional fussy spells of baby. Getting their weight checked would put needless worries to rest, or it may identify that you could have a low milk supply. If this is the case, a plan to increase your supply will be extremely valuable and may prevent low milk supply issues.

There are several factors that influence your supply of breast milk. The most common is how often your breasts are stimulated and how effectively they are being emptied. Remember, your supply is based on demand; the more frequently you empty your breasts, the more milk you will produce. Therefore skipping nursing sessions or giving baby a bottle at night will negatively impact your supply. You will notice differences in your breasts throughout your breastfeeding experience. At times, especially early in the day, they may be very full and possibly leaking, and later they will feel softer and you may not leak at all. This does not mean you aren't meeting the nutritional needs of your baby. This is how your breasts adapt to hormone changes in your body, and the feeding pattern of your baby. The best way to determine if you could have a low milk supply is to record the number of baby's feedings, wet and dirty diapers. This simple tallying of amounts, along with frequent weight checks can tell much about how your baby is breastfeeding. Frequently, a mother who makes an outpatient lactation appointment is convinced her baby isn't getting enough milk. During the appointment Baby is weighed before and after feeding at each breast. Mom is often surprised by how much milk her baby gets in a short period of time. Babies become efficient and have very effective nursing patterns as they grow.

We have lived in a culture of bottle-feeding, where the number of ounces are prominently displayed on the container. Putting trust in your breasts, where volumes are not easily visible, can be difficult. Try to abandon the thought of needing to know volumes and numbers. You need to look for positive signs in the baby, indicating they are getting enough to eat and reassuring you that your milk supply is adequate.

The following is a list of those positive signs:
- Adequate weight gaining pattern
- Meeting a minimum number of wet and dirty diapers
- Baby is content after the feeding
- Baby is satisfied between feedings
- Breasts are less full when baby is done eating
- Hearing swallows throughout the feeding

You may wonder, "How do I know if my milk supply is actually too low?" Sometimes this change can be subtle or can seem to happen suddenly overnight. Be aware of your baby's behaviors while they are nursing and any schedule or pattern changes.

Signs that Baby is not getting enough to eat would be:
- Fussy during or after their feeding
- Intermittently pulling off the breast
- Their hands are pounding at the breast during a feeding, as they are trying to massage the breast to get another let down
- Not being content, alert or sleeping after feedings
- Having few wet and dirty diapers
- Having shorter intervals between feedings
- Baby is waking to feed during the night when before they slept through the night
- You do not hear as many swallows

- Baby is overall more fussy
- Poor weight gain

Again, remember nearly every woman is capable of making enough milk for their baby. Getting a weight check on your baby may put all your worries to rest. Worrying about a milk supply can simply make you anxious for no reason. If it becomes necessary to begin a plan to increase your milk supply, your lactation consultant will be particularly helpful in determining what is needed.

Certain conditions may give you a reason for having a low milk supply. Next we will discuss these reasons.

Chapter 29: What are some reasons I might not produce enough milk?

Now you know the signs in baby that tell you the differences between actual and perceived low milk supply. The next step is to identify some possible reasons you could be struggling with your supply. You may be working hard to get your milk established, or you may be dealing with a supply that was more than adequate but now has decreased. Either way, it's important to identify the cause of this as soon as possible. Following are some situations or conditions that may be potential reasons for low milk supply. It's best to be aware of these so you can be on the lookout for any possible problems. Dealing with a low milk supply sooner rather than later can make a great difference in how long it takes to rebuild your supply.

Lactation Consultants have often considered that infertility may play a part in low milk supply. The thought is "if you're hormonally balanced for pregnancy, you should be hormonally balanced for lactation." Usually the cause of your infertility will play a more important role than simply infertility itself. If you have been diagnosed with a primary hormonal imbalance, there is potential for this imbalance to interfere with adequate breast development needed to support full lactation; or interfere with the process itself. I wouldn't consider this to be the first reason for low milk supply; however, you may think of it as a risk factor.

Polycystic Ovarian Syndrome (PCOS) is an endocrine disorder in which a woman has an imbalance in female hormones. Some common symptoms include:

- Menstrual disorders with heavy and frequent periods; or few to no periods at all
- Infertility
- Persistent acne
- Excessive hair growth on the body
- Tendency for centrally located obesity
- Insulin resistance which may lead to type 2 Diabetes
- Infrequent ovulation and endometriosis
- Brown patches of skin around the neck, under arms and groin area

There are a few theories of how PCOS leads to low milk supply. If symptoms occur at the time of puberty, normal breast development may not occur. The hormonal imbalance that causes irregular menstrual cycles and ovulation may interfere with normal milk production.

Gastric bypass is another possible red flag for low milk production. Gastric bypass surgically reduces the size of a stomach and bypasses the top portion of the small intestine. This surgery results in a drastic reduction of calories eaten each day. While this helps you lose weight, the procedure also affects the body's ability to absorb some nutrients. It is generally recommended by physicians to prevent becoming pregnant for two years following gastric bypass surgery. During this time of reduced caloric intake and restricted diet, the person is metabolizing mostly fat. This makes it difficult to consume enough essential nutrients and calories to support pregnancy and lactation. If a woman has become pregnant and is breastfeeding during this time of drastic caloric reduction, her poor nutrition can affect the quality and quantity of breast milk. Nutritional supplements, which can be helpful, are referred to in chapter 6.

Most mothers who have had breast surgeries can produce milk. However, there can be some degree of variance to just how much milk they will produce. Depending upon the type and reason for breast surgery, there may be little or no effect on breastfeeding. This topic was explained in detail previously in the beginning of this guide, but let's take a brief look at this topic again.

Breast augmentation or breast implants usually do not present problems for milk production and supply. If your primary reason for getting implants was that you had very small breasts, however, you may have insufficient glandular tissue, which could affect breastfeeding. Glandular tissue is milk-making tissue and is responsible for a large part of the production process. Even though you may be a small chested woman, if you experienced an increase in breast size during pregnancy, you will be very capable of producing plenty of milk for your baby.

Women with breast reduction surgery will find this procedure potentially more challenging on their milk supply. Breast reduction surgery actually removes tissue and disturbs the pathways of milk ducts and sinuses. This may cause problems with actual removal of the milk, as the pathways are no longer aligned. Every woman is different, so her milk supply can also be different. If you've had breast reduction surgery, I suggest you speak with a Lactation Consultant early for guidance as you begin to breastfeed. This will help you have a more successful outcome.

Some breast abnormalities may have a negative impact on milk production. If your breasts barely matured during puberty, lack fullness in all or parts of the breast, or are tubular shaped, there could be an effect on your supply. Tubular shaped breasts result from development being halted before reaching maturity. Often there is a wider space between the breasts, usually greater than two inches, and the breast appearance is long and cylindrically shaped with nipples pointing down. One of the most telling features of poor milk production is the lack of breast fullness during pregnancy and few breast changes during early lactation.

If you had a large blood loss during delivery, or a postpartum hemorrhage, you may have low hemoglobin. Hemoglobin is a protein in red blood cells that carries oxygen, a very important task. If your hemoglobin is low, called anemia, it may take longer for your milk to come in or you may make less volume. You may need the extra stimulation of pumping or you may find herbal supplements to be helpful. I will discuss herbal supplements in the upcoming chapters.

Estrogen hormone birth control pills or Depo Provera injection may also impact your milk supply and may shorten your length of breastfeeding. Progestin-only contraceptives are the preferred method for breastfeeding mothers when something hormonal is desired. For most mothers, progestin-only forms of contraception do not cause problems with milk supply if started at least 6-8 weeks after delivery. It's recommended that any estrogen-containing contraceptive be avoided until your baby is at least six months old and taking solid foods.

If you have been diagnosed with low thyroid levels, you have a condition called Hypothyroidism. This is when the thyroid gland does not make sufficient hormone amounts for the very important function of regulating body metabolism. One symptom of hypothyroidism is infertility. Most women have already been diagnosed and treated prior to lactation. However, as thyroid levels frequently change with pregnancy and breastfeeding, it is best to get your levels checked if your suspect a low thyroid level could be interfering with your milk supply.

I've primarily discussed "Mom reasons" for low milk supply, but there can be "Baby reasons" as well. Poor stimulation to the breast is one of the biggest reasons for low milk production or a delay in milk production. When the baby isn't stimulating the mother's breasts effectively, her prolactin hormone level fails to rise. The prolactin hormone tells your body how much milk to make. If the hormone level is not elevated by frequent and efficient feedings, your body gets a weak message leading to low milk supply.

Here are important signs to watch for when nursing your baby:

- Make sure your baby is being productive and sucking effectively while nursing.
- Baby has to coordinate using their tongue, jaw, cheeks, lips and their facial muscles, which can be difficult, so watch for signs of good movement and coordination of these muscles when nursing.
- Baby can be very sleepy while they are first gaining weight and some remain sleepy until they have gained back to their birth weight. Keep them actively nursing so you are feeling a strong pulling and tugging. Do not let them "comfort suck" only.

- Be sure your baby has a good, deep latch. Latches that are painful and too shallow do not stimulate well.
- Have your nurse, knowledgeable health care provider, or lactation consultant assesses a feeding to be sure your baby is effectively removing the milk.

Another possible reason for low milk supply may be that your baby is tongue-tied. This is a condition, which causes decreased mobility of the tongue due to a tight frenulum. The frenulum is the membrane connecting the underside of the tongue to the floor of the mouth. If this membrane is too tight and located too close to the tip of the tongue, your baby will have limited movement leading to decreased stimulation to the breast.

If you are using a breast pump regularly or are pumping and bottle feeding, be sure you have an effective pump. You should have your breast pump checked out by a lactation consultant, especially if it is old or borrowed. Pump pressures, cycling and efficiency vary from pump to pump. Pressures above 225-250 mm Hg negative pressure sometimes cause pain. Pressures below 150 mm Hg may be too low and ineffective. Breast pumps should cycle 45-55 times per minute, which mimics the rate of baby's sucking. Knowing you have a pump with the correct pressure range and cycles will help insure adequate stimulation. Gauges that measure pressure are relatively inexpensive and can be purchased at a hardware store or you can ask your local lactation consultant for assistance.

My hope is this list may help you pinpoint the problem causing your low milk supply. After you have identified your circumstance, you can make a plan to establish more milk, or return your supply to its previous volume. What should your plan include? How do you reverse your situation? Let's take a look at some interventions that might turn your situation around.

Chapter 30: Can I correct my problem and increase my low milk supply?

It's important to identify the cause for your decreased milk supply; remember nearly all of these problems can be corrected. So don't panic, your situation is quite reversible.

Most of the time low milk supply originates with poor breast stimulation. Whether the problem is to modify your baby's nursing pattern, sucking behavior, or his infrequent feeding schedule, the first thing to do is provide more stimulation to your breasts. If your baby can't provide this, a breast pump must provide it.

Stimulation is most effective coming from your baby; however, relying on baby alone might be the cause of your low milk supply. Now you must look to a high quality and effective breast pump to provide the extra stimulation. Using a breast pump is not always the warmest experience, but pumping may be exactly what is needed to give your body the message to increase production. More stimulation is equal to more milk, plain and simple.

I suggest pumping after as many breastfeeding sessions as possible. Be sure to not exhaust yourself, this won't help your situation. Many moms choose not to pump in the middle of the night; however this is when you will likely get the most volume. Use your judgment and common sense for what will work best for you. Try and relax when you're pumping. Watching the amount in the bottles and worrying about "how much you're getting" will do little to increase your supply. In fact, you may pump less when you are constantly looking at how much you're pumping instead of relaxing. Some moms find using a hands-free bra helpful. A hands-free bra supports the flanges and containers, freeing up your hands while you pump. This allows you to continue with other activities, like reading a book or surfing the web while you pump. It can be a great distraction!

As your baby gets older, and becomes more aware of their surroundings, they are easily distracted which leads to shorter feedings. With interruptions such as siblings playing, the dog barking or Daddy coming home from work, your baby may decide they are done eating before they have adequately stimulated or emptied your breasts. If you think this may be occurring too often, consider breastfeeding in a quiet environment whenever possible. Baby will be more focused, nurse more effectively, and nurse for longer periods of time. Your supply should go up as this keeps baby more productive. The enjoyment of quiet time with just the two of you is an added bonus!

Another intervention that I've seen work quite well is super switch nursing. This involves switching breasts several times during the feeding session. Watch the baby's sucking effort while they are nursing. Switch to the other breast as soon as the sucking begins to slow down, you no longer hear swallows or baby becomes distracted. Repeating this 2-3 times during the feeding increases breast stimulation and let down. Babies often get more milk by super switch nursing.

If your baby is taking solid foods, be sure you are breastfeeding first before your baby receives their solids. Babies are usually hungry and thirsty at mealtime. When they breastfeed first they are more aggressive when they nurse, as opposed to already being satisfied by their meal. A baby who is thirsty and hungry will put more effort into their nursing session therefore proving more stimulation and increasing your supply.

Remember, techniques used to increase milk will be most effective once you've targeted the cause. Many times there is not one single cause, therefore trying more than one of these interventions will likely improve your situation. Give yourself some time for these measures to become effective. Most of them do not work overnight, so have patience. The more you worry, the longer it may take to increase your supply. Along with the interventions mentioned, sometimes adding certain foods to your diet may also help increase your supply. Let's look at some of the more common foods that can have a positive effect on your supply.

Chapter 31: What foods can I eat that would help increase my milk supply?

Foods that have lactation-promoting properties are called lactogenic foods or galactagogues. You may run across these fancy words in your research. You will likely read that there are varying degrees of help provided by these foods; all the way from "amazing" to "not helpful at all". Some women can increase their milk supply simply by adding particular foods to their diet. Generally these foods can be found at your local grocery store and are easy to include in your daily diet. The following is a list of some foods that may help you make more milk:

Avocado - An avocado is high in fat, fiber, vitamins C and K and a good source of the mineral Potassium. This is a valuable food to vegetarians and vegans. Because fatty meats, fish and dairy products are eliminated from their diet, avocados will provide the fat needed.

Brown rice - Unprocessed rice contains complex carbohydrates, which provide energy. Researchers believe brown rice increases serotonin levels in the brain. Serotonin regulates moods and sleep and stimulates prolactin secretion; which are all great for a breastfeeding mother.

Coconut oil - Coconut oil contains large amounts of Lauric Acid, a powerful anti-microbial fatty acid that protects the baby's immune system. Pregnant and nursing mothers who eat coconut oil increase the quality of the environment in the womb as well as the quality of their breast milk. Coconut oil is easy to use and can be substituted for butter in your daily diet. I have suggested to mothers the use of coconut oil on sore nipples, and as an anti-fungal with thrush, and have seen good results using it for both.

Dried fruits - Fruits like figs, dates and apricots are high in fiber, vitamins A and C, potassium and calcium. These fruits also contain tryptophan, which naturally boost prolactin levels.

Papaya - Thought to have enzymes and phytochemicals that enhance breast tissue. Phytochemicals are compounds that occur naturally in plants. Papaya can be used as a natural sedative helping with let down.

Salmon - A great source of omega 3 fatty acids. These fatty acids improve your overall nutrition so you can produce the hormones necessary for milk production. Breast milk contains essential fatty acid (EFA). When a mother consumes more EFA in her diet she can have a higher fat content in her milk. Eating fish three times a week should have you covered. To avoid fish high in mercury, eat salmon and halibut instead of tuna or swordfish, which contain more belly fat to retain mercury.

Spinach - A good source of calcium, iron, Vitamin K, A, and foliate. Dark leafy green vegetables contain phytoestrogens. Phytoestrogens are believed to promote breast tissue health and lactation.

Steel cut oats - Oatmeal helps you relax; which releases oxytocin, a key hormone for lactation. Overall, oats are a very healthy food. It's recommended you skip the instant oatmeal and instead choose the less processed oat. The more whole grains they have, the more protein and minerals they contain.

Getting enough fluids in your diet will also help with milk production. It can be difficult keeping track of how much you've had to drink throughout the day. Women have a variety of ways they keep track of their fluids. Some drink every time they sit down to breastfeed, others will fill a half-gallon container in the morning with the goal to finish this by bedtime. The "millennium moms" keep track of how much they drink by using an app on their smart phone. There are apps designed to keep track of baby's feedings, wet and dirty diapers, and also record how much mom is drinking. Any method that reminds you to drink will be beneficial.

It is generally recommended to drink 64 ounces, or about one half gallon per day. One way to know if this is enough for you is to notice the color of your urine. When you urinate, the color should be pale yellow or clear. If your urine is dark yellow or amber, you are not drinking enough. For most women, drinking more water than recommended will have no effect on increasing your milk supply. I have talked about good nutrition throughout the entire book; your fluids are a large part of your overall nutrition.

Sometimes the type of water you are drinking can make an impact on your milk supply. The pH of your water may be important to your overall health and your milk production. In chemistry, pH measures a hydrogen ion concentration. This measure will vary from acid to alkaline or base.

- Acid - pH of less than 7
- Alkaline or base - pH of greater than 7
- Neutral - pH of 7

Typically, pure water has a pH that is neutral and often used as a reference point for acids and bases. Water can have a pH ranging from 6.5 to 8.5. Water with a pH of less than 6.5 is considered acidic and may contain copper, iron, lead, manganese and zinc. Numerous articles suggest you will have better health when your body is more alkaline.

For those of you who are avid bottled water drinkers, here is a list of popular brands of bottled waters and their pH range. Keep in mind that a pH of 8 and above is the recommended range for good health:

Water with a pH of 7- Arrowhead Water, Crystal Geyser Water, Deep Park Water, Eldorado Springs Water, Supermarket Spring Water

Water with a pH of 7.5 - Biota water, Fiji Water, Whole Foods 365 Water, Zephyrhills Water

Water with a pH of 7.9 - Eden Springs Water

Water with a pH of 8 - Deep Rock Water, Evamore Water

Water with a pH of 10 - Filtered Ionized Alkaline Water you make with your own Water Ionizer.

I have only included those brands, which have a pH of 7 or more. For the full content of this study and to see where your favorite water may fall, go to: http://www.comfytummy.com/tag/ph/#ixzz2QpnsKOxQ. I would encourage you to view the entire list, I was very surprised myself.

Foods on this list are overall good nutritious foods which also support the chemistry your body needs for lactation. Focus your diet on nutrient-dense foods; remember you are still "eating for two". Be aware of the type of water you're drinking as well. This is not the time for dieting to lose those extra few pounds. This is a time to focus on you and on baby; providing them with the most wonderful gift a mother could give, your nutritious breast milk.

What if adding these foods to your diet did not improve your supply? There are some herbal supplements you may find helpful.

Chapter 32: What herbals might help increase my milk supply?

When researching herbals and breastfeeding you will find many pages of website options, which can be confusing. Cultural attitudes about herbals and their usage in prevention, cures and overall health, are rapidly changing. Science is discovering more about herbals and their place in today's world. In this chapter I will focus on specific herbals I have personally worked with for several years; herbals that have proven to be very successful for increasing milk supply.

Generally speaking, using a combination herbal supplement will work better than a single stand-alone herb. Fenugreek is one of the most common stand-alone herbs used for low milk supply; however its effectiveness is questionable. Some women have some increase in their supply when using fenugreek, however I like better results than "some women, with some increase". Let's look at what these herbs do for breastfeeding and then examine some combinations of herbal products that may help you.

Alfalfa - The leaves and flowers make a nutritious tea that stimulates your appetite, aids digestion, and increases breast milk. Do not use alfalfa if you have lupus or another autoimmune disorder, as it may worsen symptoms. Do not use this if you are on a blood thinner, as this may thin your blood even further.

Blessed Thistle - This increases breast milk and gives an emotional uplift. The taste is bitter, so most women choose to take it in pill form. It works well when combined with fenugreek.

Fennel Seed - This herb helps to increase milk supply. It is also an herb that relieves heartburn, gas, and colic, upset stomach and improves digestion. Drinking fluids containing fennel will help you and baby.

Fenugreek - One of the oldest documented herbs used to increase milk supply for both humans and dairy cows. It is also used to flavor imitation maple syrup. The seeds are known for increasing breast milk. Fenugreek is also a popular spice used in East Indian cooking. The seeds also help with digestion; therefore drinking tea containing fenugreek will be beneficial to you and baby.

Goat's Rue - Comes from the same family of herbals as fenugreek. The leaves stimulate development of breast tissue, and it's one of the most potent herbs to increase breast milk. This is a good herbal to use if you have PCOS as it has anti-diabetic properties. Goat's Rue is also used to increase breast size in women who are not breastfeeding.

Nettle - Is a rich source of iron, calcium and folic acid. It supports the kidneys and adrenals, and is considered an anti-diabetic and diuretic. It supports thyroid function and increases breast milk.

Here are some combination herbal products... I have found these to be quite effective and have witnessed very good results with hundreds of women:

More Milk Plus and More Milk Plus Special Blend made by MotherLove Herbal Company. More Milk Plus is a combination of herbals consisting of fenugreek seed, blessed thistle, nettle, and fennel seed. It comes in a tincture or pill form.

More Milk Plus Special Blend is the same product with the addition of goat's rue. I usually recommend using More Milk Plus Special Blend if your milk is just coming in or if you did not have any breast changes during your pregnancy. Both products contain non-GMO soy lecithin, modified vegetable cellulose, coconut oil. They also do not contain any milk, dairy, egg, fish, shellfish, tree nuts, peanuts, wheat, or gluten and all the herbs are Certified Organic. Motherlove also makes a great nipple cream.

Nursing Time Tea by Fairhaven Health. This is an all-natural herbal stimulant designed to help nursing mothers increase their milk supply and soothe digestion of both mother and baby. Nursing Time Tea contains alfalfa, anise seed, blessed thistle, fennel seed and goat's rue. It enhances the quantity, quality and availability of milk. It has also been known to alleviate digestive problems, including gas and colic. This is a loose-leaf tea, as all you tea-lovers know, herbal tea leaves need room to expand to properly transfer and release all their nutrients. A loose-leaf tea is always a better option than a tea bag.

We serve this tea to mothers on the mother/baby unit at the hospital and explain the benefits to them. The tea is offered to those who have a history of low milk supply, breast surgeries or have a baby in the Neonatal Intensive Care Unit. For mothers of premature babies, it is especially important to pump as much milk for their baby as soon as possible. Premature and sick babies need that colostrum! Your colostrum is so valuable to your baby. The stem cells in your colostrum are abundant and irreplaceable. Making more milk by drinking tea is critical, so drink away ladies; this will benefit both of you.

It is possible for these herbal products to increase your milk supply, especially coupled with the extra stimulation of a breast pump, and the addition of the foods mentioned in chapter 4. There is still one more option for you. Malunggay or Moringa might be the answer. It has helped thousands of women all over the world; yes the world!

Chapter 33: What choices are there other than combination herbals?

When I talk with mothers about their low milk supply, I try to mention all the options available to them. I talk about what I've personally seen while working with hundreds of women in similar situations. Chapter 30 covers what you can do about stimulation and quality nursing time, chapter 31 lists some foods you may improve milk production and chapter 32 discusses the use of combination herbal supplements to help increase your milk supply. Now we will discuss one of the most powerful supplements I've ever used, Malunggay or Moringa.

Try to imagine a tree so powerful it's known around the world as "The Miracle Tree" and "The Tree of Life". Envision a tree where virtually every part of it can be used for the good of humanity. This tree literally saves lives. Moringa oleifera is the name of this life-changing tree. The Moringa oleifera tree is native to the Himalayas in Northwest India, but it also grows in dry, sandy soil areas with tropical weather conditions such as Africa, South Asia and South America. This fast-growing, drought resistant tree tolerates poor soil conditions. The tree itself holds large amounts of water in its roots and trunk, which is why it thrives through droughts.

There are over 90 known nutrients in the Moringa leaf. This number is impressive alone, but even more amazing is that the nutrients are present in large amounts. It's very unique to have a single plant that contains large amounts of multiple nutrients. Usually fruits and vegetables will have one or two valuable nutrients.

Here are some nutritional features of the Moringa leaf:

- 3 times more iron than found in spinach
- 3 times more potassium than found in a banana
- 4 times more calcium than found in milk
- 4 times more vitamin A than found in carrots
- 7 times more vitamin C than found in oranges
- 46 antioxidants
- 36 anti-inflammatories
- Omegas 3,6,and 9
- Contains 20 amino acids, including all 9 essential amino acids that our bodies only get from food sources.

Not only is the amount of nutrients in the leaves impressive, but also 100 % of this tree is used. The leaves, stem, fruit and seeds of the tree are all edible. The root can be used to make healing and wellness teas. The seeds are squeezed for cooking oil and also to heal wounds and sores. The "press" or leftovers from squeezing the seeds are used for water purification. The crushed leaves are a cooking spice and the seeds are fried and eaten like nuts. There are literally hundreds of uses for all parts of this tree.

For centuries cultures around the world have known the many benefits of Moringa and have been using it to help fight dysentery, yellow fever and malnutrition. Nothing has been more effective for fighting malnutrition in third world countries than the use of Moringa. The Discovery Channel created a documentary on the Moringa oleifera tree. Portions of this video can be viewed on YouTube. I highly suggest you take the time to view this video; it's incredible. It describes the use of Moringa in various areas of the world. For example, in Senegal, West Africa they give Moringa to pregnant women throughout their pregnancy and while they are breastfeeding to help achieve the best nutritional outcomes for mom and baby.

Many organizations are researching Moringa and its effects in the world. Moringa, or Malunggay as it's also called, is being researched by The National Science Foundation and the National Geographic Society.

Dr. Monica Marcu, author of the book, "Miracle Tree", is a clinical pharmacologist and writes: "This is the most exciting tree of our world". Lowell Fuglie, director of Church World Services states: "If I were to go out and design a tree which would be of maximum benefit to mankind, I'd be hard pressed to do better than the Moringa tree." I think this says it all.

A colleague and dear friend of mine began searching for answers for women with low milk supply. She is an amazing Lactation Consultant who loves to do research, thinks outside the box and is continuously expanding her learning. She always wondered if the answer to low milk supply was related to something lacking in the mother's diet, more specifically, a nutritional insufficiency. She set out on a mission to find something natural and safe with no side effects. Although this sounds like a tall order, her persistence paid off. She found the answer in Moringa.

Moringa products can be extremely beneficial to women with low milk supply. We have seen various forms of Moringa actually 'save the day' for some mothers. I have a theory as to why Moringa works so well; I feel everyone's daily diet is lacking in some nutrients. I tell mothers their diet is like a piece of Swiss cheese; it's full of holes with some being bigger than others. These holes represent specific nutrients that are lacking in their diet. Moringa as a dietary supplement fills those holes. When I look at my own diet, I couldn't tell you if I take in the recommended daily intake of vitamins A and C, or enough zinc or manganese. Do you know if your diet has met all the recommended daily allowances of all the nutrients? Chances are you don't. Using Moringa to 'fill the holes' will allow your body a full complement of daily nutrients needed to make enough breast milk for your baby. There are 4 different versions of Moringa to help with your milk supply. Let's look at each of them:

***Go-Lacta*®** - Moms around the world have turned to Go-Lacta® to increase their milk production. Made from the leaves of the Malunggay tree (moringa oleifera), it's the natural way to help you increase the amount of breast milk you produce. Each capsule is 350 mg. If you are dealing with a large deficit, I suggest taking 3 capsules 3 times a day until your supply has increased to meet the needs of your baby. Once you have achieved this, you can decrease the amount of capsules you are taking. Most women decrease to 3 per day. You may need a more gradual decrease, since every mother is different.

Zija - Also known as SmartMix. Zija is packed with Moringa's 90+ verifiable, vitamins, minerals, vital proteins, antioxidants, omega oils, and other benefits. Zija is a powder packet containing over 3,000 mg of Moringa. It was formulated to be quickly digested. For best results, take one packet first thing each morning, on an empty stomach. SmartMix is 100% natural, Halal and Kosher certified. Each box contains 8 packets of Moringa, so one box of Zija may be enough to give you the help you need.

Powder Moringa - Concentrated doses of Moringa can be purchased in a highly effective powder form. The potency is usually 5,000 mg per tablespoon. Most women take this dose 1-2 times per day, but beware; the taste is not terribly palatable. I have personally taken all of these Moringa products and this powder version did not taste good. In addition, it was more difficult to mix. The best way to consume this product is to mix it well with a smoothie or juice. You will need to shake it vigorously and drink it quickly, but it will be worth the effort due to its potency.

Tea - Moringa is available in tea form as well. I wouldn't necessarily recommend this form of Moringa to help with low milk supply. The tea form usually has a smaller dose of Moringa available therefore it is not as effective. It may however, be useful to help maintain an adequate milk supply.

Whatever form of Moringa you chose, you will likely see your milk supply increase. You will also feel better as your body receives the total nutrition to help your supply. As with all supplements, discuss taking them with your health care provider. My coworkers and I have been using these herbals to help mothers for years. I know Neonatologists and Pediatricians who love Moringa because it provides basic nutrition for mother. It contains no stimulants or caffeine and it is bioavailable, meaning when it enters your circulation, it has an immediate effect on the body. The body recognizes it as something it needs and therefore is immediately absorbed.

Malunggay is one of the most unique herbal supplements I've ever worked with. Its nutrition is so powerful it's hard to beat. One of the best advantages of using Moringa is simply for its nutrition. Anyone can take it! It will only increase milk production if your breasts are being stimulated by nursing or pumping. That's why non-lactating people can take Moringa, old and young, men and women, nursing and non-nursing. I urge you to view the documentary on YouTube, read about Moringa and talk to your health care provider to see if a Moringa product might be right for you. I think you will be pleasantly surprised.

Human milk production is an amazing process. Your body is constantly tailoring your milk supply to meet the exact needs of your baby. However, when this process seems like it's not working, as it should, the information included in this book is your guide. Increasing their milk supply is a real concern for many breastfeeding women. I have given you some possible reasons for your low milk supply and solid interventions to help you increase your supply. I've given several options to choose from so that you can find the best solution for you.

Every woman has dreams and goals over the course of their breastfeeding experience. Everyone would like to see those goals met and those dreams come true. I wish the best for you as you increase your milk supply and continue to meet your personal breastfeeding goals.

Chapter 34: I wasn't expecting this, what happens now?

Having a premature or sick baby isn't anything that's planned by any means. Parents have valid questions and concerns spinning around in their heads such as; "I'm not ready for this baby.", "What did I do wrong?" "What do I do now?", and most of all, "Is my baby going to be alright?" You may have had an uncomplicated, problem-free pregnancy that changed very quickly. This has left you little time to process your situation. Due to warnings during your pregnancy, some of you might have expected an early birth, or perhaps have experienced this before. It's still a difficult situation. Some parents feel cheated by not experiencing what they had always dreamed of, a healthy, full term baby.

Remember, 40% of premature births occur for no known reasons. But some women may be considered high risk based on their obstetrical history or the presence of known risk factors.

Here are some recognized maternal risk factors to be aware of:

- Poor maternal nutrition
- History of a preterm birth
- Women either early or late in their reproductive years
- African-American women
- Short spacing between births
- If baby has a birth defect
- Multiples; twins or triplets or more
- Hypertension or high blood pressure

Book Series #6: When Unexpected Situations Separate You and Baby

- Vaginal bleeding during pregnancy
- Abnormal amounts of amniotic fluids; too much or too little
- Anxiety and depression
- Tobacco, street drugs or excessive alcohol during pregnancy
- Maternal infections

There are varying levels of prematurity. The earlier the baby is born, the more severe the health problems they are likely to have.

A very low birth weight, VLBW, infant is called a micro preemie. These babies are born weighing less than 1.7 pounds, 800 grams or born before 26 weeks gestation. They have long hospital stays in the NICU, as they are extremely fragile and have uncertain outcomes. Each additional day a baby can remain in their mother's womb may mean the difference between life and death during those second trimester weeks.

The micro preemie baby has very thin skin with visible veins and their eyes may be fused shut. They will need intravenous or IV lines for extra fluids, and respiratory support in the form of a ventilator, which breathes for them. Some babies are able to breathe on their own, but will need assistance of continuous positive airway pressure or a CPAP machine. They will be attached to machines that provide continuous monitoring of their vital signs.

If your baby is born a micro preemie, you can expect to postpone breastfeeding for quite some time. These VLBW babies are too immature to eat from a bottle or from the breast. You will spend your time working to bring in a full milk supply for your baby. This will need to happen using a breast pump. The sooner you begin pumping the better your supply will be. You can expect to pump your breasts 8 times every 24 hours, as this would be a full term baby's feeding pattern.

The preterm baby is born between 26 and 34 weeks gestation. Their weight ranges from 3.3 to 5.5 pounds or 1,500 to 2,500 grams. Characteristics of a preterm baby depend upon their weeks of gestation and their birth weight.

Most of the babies born within this gestation period will have abnormal breathing patterns. Some will require ventilators or CPAP machines as described above. They will have low muscle tone, less body fat, soft cartilage around their ears, and thin, shiny skin that remains transparent like the micro preemie. They have problems coordinating their sucking, swallowing and breathing patterns. It is for this reason many preemie babies have difficulty eating and will require tube feedings. A nasogastric or NG tube is inserted in their nose and goes into their stomach for feedings. It will take time for them to coordinate the skills for successful breastfeeding. This is normal, so try to be patient with them as they are learning.

A late preterm baby is born after 34 weeks and before 37 weeks gestation. These babies are frequently healthier than the preterm infant, but can also be affected by complications. Often their appearance is similar to a full term baby, only smaller. Although the late preterm may not have the physical characteristics of the micro preemie or preterm baby, they are still at risk for complications. These babies are likely to suffer from respiratory distress, difficulty with feedings, have unstable blood sugars and difficulty regulating their body temperatures.

A term baby is born anytime after 37 weeks gestation. Even full term babies can be sick and need to be in an NICU setting. Full term babies may still have breathing problems, unstable blood sugars, restricted growth, cardiac problems or infections when they are born. Fortunately, the majority of full term babies are born healthy.

There are many potential situations causing premature birth. It is vital you take good care of yourself as soon as you know you are pregnant. Living healthy before, during and after a pregnancy will give you the best chance for a carrying your baby to term, leading to successful breastfeeding. It is critical to have your baby as close to your due date as possible. Having a premature baby is a stressful situation for the entire family, especially if they are a micro-preemie or very ill baby. Take care of yourself, and try to stay pregnant as long as possible. This decision could literally make a life-changing difference for you and your baby.

Chapter 35: My baby is early and so very small, how can I help them?

Having a very premature or critically ill child can put the family into crisis. Overwhelming feelings of confusion and helplessness are frequently shared by parents of these babies. The future is unknown and being in unfamiliar territory can produce anxiety as well. Breastfeeding these infants can present a whole new set of challenges. It is possible that some of you will become discouraged with the process and want to give up at some point along the way. While there may be unexpected challenges and disappointing moments, the benefits you alone can provide to your baby will be worth your efforts. This chapter was written to help calm your fears and address what you can do as you grieve your dream and accept your situation.

One thing you can do for your preterm baby is to experience the touching and bonding time of skin-to-skin. Being close to you is a newborn's natural habitat and the one in which they are meant to thrive. Here is a story of how skin-to-skin began and started helping premature babies.

Dr. Nils Bergman is considered by many to be the "founder" of skin-to-skin, or as he calls it, Kangaroo Mother Care. Dr. Bergman was the Medical Superintendent and District Medical Officer at Manama Mission, Zimbabwe. Here he developed and implemented Kangaroo Mother Care for premature infants. He introduced Kangaroo Mother Care to South Africa in 1995. The results were amazing and after only 5 years, this became the official policy for care of preemie babies in hospitals of the Western Cape Province. This demonstrates how important skin-to-skin can be in the case of a premature baby.

Dr. Bergman says all the basic needs of a baby are being met by doing skin-to-skin. Their need for oxygen, warmth, nutrition and protection can be provided, even as early as 28 weeks. Of course, doing skin-to-skin will largely depend on your baby's physical condition. Skin-to-skin should be done as early and frequently as possible and for as long as possible.

I have discussed skin-to-skin in depth already but here is a summary of the benefits of skin-to-skin to both you and baby:

- Stabilizes Baby's heart rate and body temperature
- Regulates breathing pattern with fewer apnea episodes
- Stabilized oxygen levels
- Decreases stress hormones for both Mom and Baby
- Better bonding between baby and parents
- Faster brain maturation and development
- Improves weight gaining pattern
- More successful breastfeeding and more milk production
- Parents feel more involved with the care of their baby
- Parents have less anxiety and depression
- Which all lead to going home earlier!

The milk production process begins right away after your baby is born even when born prematurely. For that reason it is extremely important to begin pumping right away, even though you may be concerned and making decisions about the care of you baby.

Here are some of the many documented reasons for getting the breastfeeding process started early.

Enteromammary response - An enteromammary response is a system of immunity that puts antibodies into breast milk to protect Baby from their environment. When a mother's body touches her preterm baby through skin-to-skin contact, her body will detect and make specific antibodies to fight infectious agents in the baby's environment; whether that environment is in New York, New Delhi, New Zealand, or the Neonatal

Intensive Care Unit. These specific antibodies will be present in her milk and will help protect her baby from local germs they encounter. For this reason NICU babies have fewer infections when they have their own mother's milk.

Colonization of the intestines - Your baby's gut is sterile at the time of their birth. Within hours after birth they are exposed to a non-sterile environment. As this happens, they begin to populate microorganisms. This begins in their mouth and travels the length of their intestinal system where colonization begins. The influence of these microorganisms depends on what the gut is exposed to first. If the baby's gut is first exposed to infant formula, they will take in mainly bacteroids or bacteria. If on the other hand, the first exposure is to Mother's breast milk, they will be introduced to bifidobacterium. This bifidobacterium creates a more harmonious environment in the intestinal tract. The first bacteria exposure sets the stage for the environment in baby's gut for the long haul. Breast milk and even donor breast milk will set baby up for a healthier digestive system.

Colostrum - This is the first milk your body produces. As mentioned in previously, colostrum contains antibodies to protect a newborn against disease. Colostrum is also low in fat and high in protein, which is exactly what a newborn needs for their first feedings. Colostrum also contains stem cells, a lot of them! There are 50,000 stem cells in one milliliter, or 1/5th of a teaspoon of colostrum. This is an incredible life-changing amount. These stem cells are undifferentiated, meaning they have not yet been told what type of cell to become. The baby's body will determine what type of cell is most needed and the stem cells will become that type of cell. It's an amazing process. Colostrum also has a laxative-effect on Baby's intestinal system, helping them to have their first stool. This stool is quite thick and can be particularly difficult for the preterm to pass. In addition, colostrum helps with nerve function and nerve cell to cell communication. This wonderful first milk also contains growth factors, which stimulate the development of the gut. In a nutshell colostrum heals, repairs and modifies the intestinal environment setting the baby up for future digestive health.

Breast milk - There are a multitude of advantages to your baby when they are receiving your breast milk. One of the biggest advantages for the preterm is less incidence of Necrotizing Enterocolitis (NEC). This condition happens when a portion of the baby's bowel tissue becomes inflamed and necrotic or dies, this occurs in approximately 7-10% of micro preemies. Breast milk also offers easier digestion for these VLBW babies, with less gas and abdominal distention. Breast milk is also the best substitution for amniotic fluid that baby floated in and at one time digested. Breastfeeding facilitates bonding and improved developmental outcomes.

Pumping - Mothers of preterm babies may have some difficulty achieving a full milk supply. One reason is that you are relying only on a breast pump, not a baby to stimulate you. When you use a breast pump there is only the action of 'suck and release'. There is less stimulation without the compression component of the breastfeeding baby. Mothers might want to perform their own breast compression while they are pumping to increase their supply. This can be especially useful while pumping for a premature baby.

Another reason for potential low milk supply may be a delay in starting to pump or infrequent pumping sessions. Your supply is based on the demand it receives; what you demand of your body, it will supply. So, if you pump only 3 times a day, you will make enough milk for 3 feedings per day, if you're lucky. Develop a pumping schedule with frequent stimulation and frequent emptying of the breast. Remember baby eats at least 8 times a day, therefore the number of pumpings should match the number of feedings.

Skin-to-skin is something only you can do to help your baby by giving warmth, food and love. When you look at your baby, you feel an instant need to provide for and parent your baby. When you do skin-to-skin you will fill this need. Giving your breast milk is another way you can parent; provide nutrition for your baby and this helps you have some control and participation with your situation. Your breast milk will help contribute to your baby's speedy journey home. Both of these interventions will foster your bond and prepare you both for a successful transition to home.

Chapter 36: What can I expect when my baby starts to breastfeed?

There are different emotions for parents when they get the green light for the first breastfeeding session. Reactions can be anything from scared to elated, and everything in between. As a Lactation Consultant, I've personally seen the importance of having realistic expectations when beginning to breastfeed your little one. Each baby is different, each phase of their growth and development is different and, of course, each mother is different.

According to Nils Bergman, breastfeeding is a brain-based behavior of the newborn. They are all born with the behavioral ability to breastfeed. However, the preterm may not be physically capable of breastfeeding due to their fragile state. Skin-to-skin is the first step to effectively stimulate the baby's brain for future breastfeeding. Even though your baby is ill or premature, their reflexes, responses and brain activity remain ready for breastfeeding.

When you first begin to breastfeed your baby, having realistic expectations will prevent you from becoming discouraged and wanting to giving up. Remember the bonding time spent and getting to know your baby is equally as important for them. Your baby is getting to know you as well.

Here are some typical nursing behaviors and things to remember for premature babies. Keep in mind that each baby is different.

Before 35 weeks gestation:
- Offer skin-to-skin before each feeding if possible. This will stimulate their brain-based behavior and prepare them for the activity of breastfeeding.

- Preterm babies don't have much stamina, so their breastfeeding attempts may be brief.
- The frequency of their breastfeeding attempts is determined by their physical condition. When Baby is able to breastfeed, it may be for only 1-2 times each day. Try not to be discouraged, these attempts will increase quickly if you continue to do skin-to-skin. Ask your baby's doctor if they are able to do skin-to-skin more often than just before breastfeeding sessions.
- Minimal sucking is common, as they are just learning the sequence of suck, swallow and breathe. This pattern takes a great deal of coordination and every baby's efforts are different.
- They will likely have a weak suck, often weaker than your breast pump. Their energy level is not very lively yet.
- The classic breastfeeding behavior of a preterm baby is erratic and unpredictable. They may have one great feeding, and then behave like it's their first time breastfeeding at the next feeding. Those preterm babies keep you guessing so try not to look at this pattern as a failure.
- An important aspect of breastfeeding your preemie baby is for you to have a full milk supply. At this time it's even beneficial for you to have an over-abundant milk supply.
- Because baby's suck is weak, getting an easy reward from an abundant supply of milk will positively reinforce even their fragile sucking behavior. They will begin to connect the dots between you, your milk, and their new method of feeding.

Older than 35 weeks gestation:
- Continue to begin feedings with skin-to-skin.
- Your baby is growing and looking more like a full term baby, however they may continue to breastfeed like a younger baby.
- Your baby will likely awaken for some of their feedings, which is a great sign they are growing up.

Book Series #6: When Unexpected Situations Separate You and Baby

- Their unpredictable breastfeeding behavior continues, however you will begin to see noticeable improvement and consistencies as they get closer in weeks to full term.
- Their suck will be stronger than when you first began to breastfeed.
- You will notice their coordination improve as they develop their suck, swallow and breathing pattern.
- You may see their endurance improve, however the ability to take an entire feeding at the breast is usually the last hurdle they cross.
- Frequently a supplemental feeding after nursing is necessary until your baby becomes stronger. As they mature, these additional feedings will decrease in frequency and amount. Eventually they will be able to consume an entire feeding at the breast, no supplements needed.
- You will continue pumping to keep your abundant supply.
- Celebrate all successes!

Term baby:

- Although your baby is full term, they are sick and will not behave like a full term baby.
- Your baby's breastfeeding behaviors can range from wonderful to uninterested and struggling.
- Full term babies may be jaundice, may have difficulty breathing or have trouble maintaining their temperature and most times will be getting IV fluids. All these problems can make them disinterested in breastfeeding. They will need time to transition and stabilize.
- Full term babies are more likely to have successful breastfeeding, but may still be inconsistent from feeding to feeding.
- Begin your feedings with skin-to-skin whenever possible.
- Full term babies can make rapid progress with breastfeeding; so be prepared for anything.
- Many moms think they don't have to pump because they have a full term baby. Because you may not have consistent emptying of

your breast by your baby, the pump will be needed to make up the difference. This assures you have a full milk supply when your baby does decide they are ready.

Having realistic expectations for you and your baby as you bond and breastfeed will help you feel competent and avoid frustration. Understanding your preterm baby's reflexes, instincts and capabilities will create realistic expectations, and will help you avoid disappointment or the feeling of failure, therefore breastfeeding starts very slowly. Your child is unique and their behavior at the breast can be unique as well. Your baby is in need of special care and that's why they are in the hospital instead of home with you. Although it may be difficult, they are where they need to be. Be patient with your baby and with yourself. Celebrate any forward progress and focus your attention on keeping your milk supply plentiful.

Chapter 37: I have so many different emotions, how can I process them?

You are likely to have an array of emotions throughout this experience, so it is important to know you're not alone. Having someone to talk with can be invaluable as you navigate through the medical terms, disappointments and the victories. In this chapter I will cover ways of coping with the emotions that accompany being separated from your baby.

Although situations vary among premature and ill babies, there are many common emotions for the parents. Having the feelings of sadness, fear and uncertainty may surprise you, when you hoped the birth of your child would bring joy and happiness. The worries, fears of the future and how helpless you feel about parenting, seem to consume your daily thoughts. If you are feeling powerless, here are some suggestions to help you cope with your situation.

Support groups bring together people who are facing similar life challenges and changes. A support group focuses on a specific situation or condition. Members of a support group will often share their experiences and give advice; this sharing will be helpful when dealing with an early or ill baby. Support can come in a variety of formats; group settings or one on one chats by telephone or the Internet. Any format will be helpful.

Regardless of how you receive it, support has many benefits.

- Gives you awareness of resources or other treatment options that may be helpful
- Others can help you look ahead to what might be new territory and better equip you to handle what lies ahead

- Help you improve your coping skills
- Reduces your anxiety or depression
- Helps you gain control and feel more empowered
- Makes you feel less isolated and lonely
- Helps to normalize you're feelings and emotions
- Sharing understanding of what you are experiencing

Ask your health care provider for recommendations and resources about a preterm situation. Every NICU should have a social worker that can offer information and resources to help you. Contacting your local library, religious facility or looking on the Internet may be a way for you to find support. I highly recommend you tap into at least one resource to help you get through this challenge. I have seen long-term friendships develop between families going through shared experiences.

Lactation Consultants receive feedback from mothers who are pumping for their hospitalized baby. What we hear is that pumping helped them stay connected to their baby, even before they were able to hold them. If you have a micro preemie or a very ill baby this may become even more important. Feelings of helplessness create a strong need to do something for your baby. When you're pumping, you're doing the most important nurturing action anyone can do for your baby. This is your greatest accomplishment; giving your baby the one thing no one else can give. Only you have the specific medicine needed for your baby; your breast milk. Be proud of that!

Remember that hospitals will do everything they can to support your breastfeeding goals. The NICU team will use all their resources to help parents see their dream become reality. They involve parents early in the care so you become knowledgeable and confident in it. The NICU staff wants you to have success with breastfeeding and milk production. The more of mother's breast milk that baby receives, the stronger and healthier they will become. Taking home a healthy baby is everyone's goal. When you keep milk production ample and are patient with yourself and your baby, you can experience successful breastfeeding even when separated. A sense of accomplishment follows when you are able to continue providing breast milk for your baby.

Journaling is a form of expression therapy and can be very useful in a variety of settings. There is increasing evidence to support journaling provides a positive impact on your physical well-being. Because you're in a stressful and demanding situation with a baby in an NICU setting, you might find journaling helpful. Recording even just a few words each day will help you remember events or milestones of your baby's stay. The days are likely to blend together and you will forget when one event ends and another begins. You might find journaling helpful to express feelings and clarify your thoughts, as your emotions may be scattered all over the place. Combine your situation with the racing postpartum hormones in your body, and you might find journaling to be just what you need.

Here are some benefits to journaling:

- Allows you to release and express thoughts and emotions
- Help you to process difficult events
- Increases focus and bring you stability and clarity
- Acts as a counselor of sorts
- Allows you to look back to see how far you've come
- Helps you sort things out allowing you to become better prepared
- Records the past; logs your baby's progress
- Gives you confidence in yourself and what you are doing for your baby
- Links you to the bigger picture of your situation and goals
- Provides self-discovery
- Journaling can provide both emotional and psychological relief.
- If you record your pumping progress and milk supply it helps you know when to contact a Lactation Consultant if your supply decreases.

Looking back on stressful and exhausting situations can be a reminder of your strength and confidence you've gained to care for your baby at home. You may find your journal is your best friend. I suggest you give it a try!

You are likely to have an array of emotions during the separation of you and your baby, so it's important to know this is normal and you're not alone. Seeking help and journaling will be healthy aspects to your experience. Also, you need the hospital to support your breastfeeding goals and to provide early involvement in your baby's care whenever possible.

You made it though the difficulties of separation and you're bringing baby home. What a wonderful, yet potentially worrisome time. As the day for coming home gets closer, instead of feeling confident and well equipped to parent, you now have doubt and uncertainty.

Chapter 38: We're going home! Will I know what to do?

Congratulations! Your baby is home. What a great accomplishment for the entire family. You have all worked hard to make this happen, especially your baby. There were many mountains to climb and hurdles to jump, but you all did it. Happiness and joy followed you home, but this monumental occasion can come with some mixed emotions as well.

For days, weeks or even months you have had Pediatricians, Neonatologists, Registered Nurses and Lactation Consultants at your disposal. You may be feeling a bit overwhelmed now that the support team isn't handy. Remember, no one knows your baby as well as you do. No one has nurtured your baby the way you have. Trust yourself, remember the skills you've learned and know that you can still ask for help. Now is when you will have the best opportunity to become emotionally connected and physically close to your baby. Enjoy every minute of this and have confidence in yourself. Everything will come together. Your baby is so lucky to have you for their parent.

If you are taking home a full term baby, you may be able to exclusively breastfeed. There might not be a need for supplementing or even for pumping, depending on how well your baby nursed while in the hospital. You should receive guidance about this at the time of discharge.

If your baby was premature you are likely taking them home before their due date. Because they are preterm, it's not likely they are exclusively breastfeeding at discharge. However, these preemie babies can surprise us.

You will likely have a feeding plan to follow if your baby will not yet take a complete feeding at your breast. If your Baby isn't taking their entire feeding at the breast, you will need to follow a three-step plan that will look something like this:

Step 1 - Continue to offer the breast first. Let Baby nurse as long as they are productively nursing. This may mean Baby is only nursing for a few minutes. When your baby becomes sleepy and is no longer nursing well, end the feeding. The biggest mistake parents make when working with a premature baby is to let them stay at the breast only "attempting" for too long a time. Their window of opportunity for a feeding is often quite short. Your baby's endurance will increase with time.

Step 2 - Supplementing your baby. When you supplement or give them additional milk after you have nursed, you are providing the extra calories they need to gain weight. Use any milk you have previously pumped for their supplement. At the time of their discharge, you should have been given guidance as to the amount of supplement your baby needs.

Step 3 - Pump after all or most feedings. This will provide the additional stimulation you are not getting from your baby. Remember, supply is based on demand; the more demand put on the breast, the greater the milk supply. The pump will now take over where your baby left off. Try to pump right after you have ended the supplement with your baby. Or, if someone is there to provide the supplement to your baby, pump right after they are done breastfeeding. This will provide more effective stimulation while your hormones are still elevated.

Babies going home from an NICU or Special Care Nursery will have a follow up appointment soon after discharge. Your baby's health care provider will want to be sure you are both doing well with this new change. Parents usually have multiple questions and concerns as they start their role as the primary care giver. I suggest you make a list of questions and bring along another person for that first appointment. You may forget to ask some questions during the visit or you may not hear everything that's said. It is an immense responsibility taking care of a premature infant and this is an important time to ask for help. If Dad cannot be the "second set of ears" at the appointment, bring a friend or relative with you.

Being home with your baby can be a completely satisfying and fulfilling time. You will be thrilled to do something more traditional; something you dreamed of or perhaps something you enjoyed with another child. Take a moment for the two of you to just hang out and be together whenever possible. Make up for the time and experiences that were lost during your separation.

Throughout your pregnancy you have dreamed about your baby and become excited in the anticipation of it all. You likely envisioned how your baby would come into the world, what their chubby little face would look like, breastfeeding them for the first time, and of course the day you bring them home. Having a premature or ill baby means the reality of those dreams might be different. Nothing can really prepare you for this, even if you've been there before. However, this doesn't mean you have to abandon the dream you've imagined, even though it is modified a bit. You can still have the breastfeeding experience you want, remember to talk with your Lactation Consultant who will guide to towards breastfeeding success.

Each family experience is unique, but there are common threads of fear, struggles, desires and victories. Those hard-fought victories will last a lifetime. You will be thankful for them every time you look at the sweet face of your precious gift.

Chapter 39: What rights do I have when I return to work?

Until recently, women had very few laws or regulations to support their decision to continue breastfeeding while returning to work. Today as legislators have brought about change, there are new laws that help working mothers who are breastfeeding. The Patient Protection and Affordable Care Act spells out guidelines for employers to follow and how they must support women and their decision to pump in the workplace.

The Affordable Care Act (ACA) was passed by Congress and signed into law by President Obama on March 23, 2010. This health insurance reform is meant to make prevention affordable and accessible for all Americans by requiring health plans to cover preventative services. A preventative service is one that shows strong scientific evidence of future health benefits. Plans can no longer charge a patient a copayment, coinsurance or deductible for these services when they are delivered by a network provider. Guidelines were developed by the Institute of Medicine that helped define a comprehensive set of preventative services. You can find a complete listing of women's preventative services covered by visiting www.hrsa.gov/womensguidelines.

Breastfeeding services covered under the Affordable Care Act include breastfeeding support, supplies and counseling. Insurance coverage for the breastfeeding mother is described as follows; "Comprehensive lactation support and counseling, provided by a trained provider, occur during pregnancy and/or in the postpartum period and include costs for renting breastfeeding equipment."

Not only did the ACA change insurance coverage for breastfeeding women, it defined what the employer must provide for the nursing mother who is returning to work. The ACA of 2010 requires all employers to provide, upon an employee's request, "reasonable break time" for her to express milk, not including time actually breastfeeding her child. A child is considered up to one year of age. The employer will need to provide a private location for pumping other than a bathroom. The employer does not have to pay her wages for these breaks. Employers with fewer than 50 employees who demonstrate hardship in complying with the law may be exempted.

The ACA law made two major changes that helped breastfeeding women. The first provided insurance coverage for preventative services of breastfeeding and the second caused the employer to comply with a new set of rules for a nursing mother who is returning to work. Section 4207 of the ACA describes and empowers all women who wish to have their breastfeeding efforts supported.

Although these changes may not cover everything, they are a beginning and will help you when you return to work. I suggest you know your rights, stand up for them, and have a plan in place before returning to work. Talk to your employer before returning, share your plan with them and address any real or potential problems that could arise. You may find it helpful to have this discussion before you go on maternity leave. Anything that will make your return to work easier and less stressful means more success. Remember there are benefits to both you and baby when you continue breastfeeding while returning to work.

Chapter 40: What are the benefits to my baby and me when I provide pumped milk?

Since 1997, the American Academy of Pediatrics (AAP) has recommended that all babies receive breast milk for a minimum of one year. These AAP guidelines continue to urge employers to provide support and a place for women to pump their milk. I've talked in depth about the benefits of breast milk to both mother and baby. These benefits don't end if your breast milk is given by a bottle. You can continue to put your baby to breast during evenings, early mornings, weekends, and whenever you and baby are together.

Benefits to Baby include:
- About 50-100 stem cells per milliliter, or 1/5th of a teaspoon are still available in mature breast milk
- Cognitive development continues
- Protecting the intestinal system
- Less chance of childhood obesity
- Less chance for Sudden Infant Death Syndrome (SIDS)
- Fewer ear infections, diarrhea and colds
- Fewer respiratory infections, especially important during the winter cold and flu season
- Higher overall IQ

Benefits to Mother include:
- Continue to burn those extra 300-500 calories each day that your body needs to produce breast milk for your baby

- Greater protection against ovarian and breast cancers
- Stronger bones
- Financial savings of approximately $300 per month by not purchasing infant formula
- Fewer days missed at work due to an ill child
- Keeping your dream alive to provide breast milk for your baby for as long as possible

Don't abandon breastfeeding altogether. There are still many benefits for both of you. Women often find pumping at work to be quite manageable. This time away from the rapid pace of work, can be a relaxing time for you. A time when you can focus your thoughts on you, your baby, the benefits of breastfeeding, and continue to feel good about what you're doing. To help you focus, have a picture of your baby attached to your breast pump. That will make pumping time seem to go quickly.

Chapter 41: What are the benefits to my employer when I pump at work?

Some employers may ask, "Why should we have an interest in how a woman chooses to feed their baby? Isn't that getting into her personal life?" While this may sound valid on the surface, encouraging women who make the choice to continue breastfeeding provides financial gain to the company. Supporting women who choose to pump at the work place helps a company retain good employees and to control costs.

Companies who provide a lactation room and or have a lactation program available to their employees will reclaim many benefits. Some of these benefits include:

- Reduction in staff turnover
- Higher job productivity, employee satisfaction and overall morale
- Obtaining the good reputation of a company who supports women and is concerned for the welfare of their employees
- Reduction in sick time or personal leave related to a sick child
- Less family health care costs because of healthier breastfed babies
- Fewer medical insurance claims because of less doctor visits for both Mom and Baby

The more new mothers who come back to work and continue to breastfeed, the more money the company can save. I suggest employers have an actual lactation area that is designed for the sole purpose of expressing breast milk. When creating a lactation room, here are a few suggestions:

- Provide a dedicated private area (not a bathroom or closet)
- Furnish the room with comfortable chairs, small tables and curtained cubicles so that more than one mother at a time can pump.
- Mother may want a refrigerator for storing expressed milk
- Electrical outlets are necessary
- A sink for hand washing and rinsing pumping equipment is essential
- Providing a hospital grade double electric breast pump would be preferred, but the employee may be responsible for providing their own pump.
- A bulletin board where mothers can post pictures of their baby, ask other mothers questions and post lactation services available in your area.

You are now an advocate for breastfeeding your baby, and may need to stand up for yourself and your baby. There may be other breastfeeding women at your workplace, who have paved the way for you. Talk with them and to your immediate manager. Ask about the lactation program at your work facility, and research any state laws available for breastfeeding mothers. When you prepare for your return to work, your employer can appreciate your open and sincere requests and will respect you for doing what's best for your baby.

Chapter 42: What do I need to be prepared for pumping at work?

In this chapter I will discuss finding the right pump for you, and establishing a pumping routine. As you get close to the time of returning to work, pumping a few times at home will help you get comfortable with the process. Remember as time goes on, you will get more efficient and pumping at work will be a simple routine. Envision yourself back at work; where will you be pumping? At what times will you be pumping? Where will you store your expressed milk? Is there another mom who is pumping, who you can go to for assistance and support? Answering these questions will help you transition more easily to your new pumping and working routine. However, first you must find the best breast pump for your needs.

Choosing the right pump for you will take some research on your part. I suggest you invest in a good quality double electric pump. A quality pump efficiently removes the milk, keeps your supply up and makes it easier for you to continue breastfeeding longer. Hospital-grade pumps are heavy-duty efficient pumps that have a rapid suck and release cycle. These pumps are double electric pumps meaning you can remove milk from both breasts at the same time. These pumps are high quality but typically too expensive to own as your personal pump. They can, however, be rented on a monthly basis.

The next option is a personal use double electric pump. These are affordable, portable and convenient for women who have an established milk supply. By the time you are going back to work, your supply should be established. Designed for a single user, these pumps are not meant for sharing. If you are planning to use your pump every day, you will likely need a double pump to keep an adequate milk supply.

The last two options include the single electric or battery operated breast pump, and the single-manual pump. The single electric pump is designed for short term or occasional use and generally only allow for one-sided pumping. The manual pump requires you to squeeze a lever or pump a piston to create the suction. This method is time consuming and tedious. Neither of these would be options for a returning-to-work pump, unless you work very few hours.

How often you are able to pump will be important to your overall goal and success. In an ideal situation, you should pump when your baby would be eating. This will keep your body's routine the same as baby's is. In your work setting, that may not always be possible and quite often this does not happen. It is, in reality, more important that you pump as many times as your baby would eat while you are gone. For instance, if you are away from your baby for three feedings, you would need to pump three times while you are away. Again, your work schedule may not allow this regularity. Explore your option and see if there are any changes or adjustments you could make to your workday. For example, if you have a private office, perhaps you could use a hands-free bra and pump while you continue working. These bras are relatively inexpensive and allow you to have both hands free so you can type, read and even eat while you are pumping. This bra has been a real lifesaver for many women.

If your workday allows fewer pumpings than your baby is eating, it will be necessary to make the most of each and every pumping. Here are some tips while you are pumping:

- Be sure you have a thorough pumping of at least 15 minutes
- Have the suction setting on the pump as high, yet as comfortable, as possible. If your suction setting is uncomfortably high you will get less milk volumes, as this can affect your letdown.
- Relax! Don't look at the volumes you are pumping. You will pump more if you don't look and put undo pressure on yourself.

- Go to your "happy place". Think of you and your baby, imagine you are nursing your baby and look at their picture. Use relaxation techniques previously learned.
- Breast compression may help as well. Breast compression is using your hand to gently massage the milk through the milk ducts. There are many videos of this on YouTube.
- Double pump for your first 10+ minutes, then switch your pump to single pumping and do some breast compression or massage to each breast for the remaining 5+ minutes. Many women find they pump more when adding breast compression to the end of each pumping.

You may feel more confident about returning to work if you already have a supply stored in your freezer. You may begin this process after your hormones are stable and your baby has regained their birth weight. By pumping the "leftovers" after your baby is done breastfeeding, you can store this pumped milk. This will allow you to safely store some extra milk without over producing. Pumping before you actually return to work also allows you to get familiar with your pump.

Before returning to work, be sure you have introduced your baby to a bottle and kept this with some regularity. By waiting until breastfeeding is going well and Baby is gaining weight, you can prevent nipple confusion for your baby and not slow your supply. Knowing your baby will take a bottle from others will help you feel more confident about returning to work. Your baby's caregiver or day care provider will appreciate this even more than you do!

Coordinate your baby's schedule, breast milk use and storage instructions with your day care provider. They will appreciate the clear guidelines and expectations. If possible your baby should be ready for a feeding once you are home. Getting a good emptying after a day of pumping will be good for your supply and comfort. If your baby is hungry before your arrival, your caregiver could tide them over with a smaller snack-size feeding.

A few helpful tips when coordinating feedings, milk storage, and schedules with your daycare provider are as follows:

- Your baby may not drink as much milk from a bottle as you think. If Baby is about 5-6 weeks of age, start out with amounts in each bottle, of 2-4 ounces. Send an extra bottle of milk if more is needed.
- Offer the milk with a slow flow nipple and don't rush the baby to finish the last drop. Breast milk digests and satisfies quickly, so forcing baby to eat more at each feeding may actually result in overfeeding.
- Provide enough filled bottles for the hours you are gone. Often 3 feedings for a normal workday are appropriate.
- There is no need to wear gloves when feeding breast milk.
- If Baby does not eat much at day care, you will have the opportunity to nurse at home and don't worry; they will regulate what they need.
- Thawed milk can be stored in the refrigerator for 24 hours so thawing it overnight for the next day works well.
- If Baby is really hungry when you pick them up from daycare, a quick nursing will make the ride home more comfortable for both of you.
- The distraction of driving home with a hungry, crying Baby in the back seat can be hazardous.

Many women find returning to work on a part-time basis very helpful, even if for the first 2-3 weeks. This allows for less stress as you ease into this new routine. If this is not an option, return one week sooner. This would allow you to split the first two weeks into part-time. Another option may be returning to return on a Wednesday or Thursday, making that week a partial workweek.

Your milk supply might need to adjust to your new schedule and you may find you don't produce as much milk at first. This is very common and usually temporary as your body adapts to this new routine. This is where having a supply in your freezer may come in handy. If you continue to pump less milk even when following these pumping tips, refer to keep reading for methods to increase your milk supply. I am confident there will be solutions that would work for you.

Women have been going back to work and successfully breastfeeding for decades. Having support at home and at work will help the process along. Talk to your employer and your day care provider to anticipate potential difficulties, and most importantly have a positive "I can do this" attitude!

Chapter 43: What is the best way to store pumped milk?

Breast milk is easy to store and when frozen can last for a very long time. There will be no need to waste a drop! You will find yourself comfortable with the routine of pumping and storing your breast milk before you know it. When pumping at work, you can store your milk in a cooler with ice packs. Plan ahead and leave milk for the next day, with your daycare provider, when you pick up your baby.

As you research the storage time of expressed breast milk, you are likely to find slightly different answers. I like to use one quick and easy rule; freshly pumped breast milk can store at room temperature for 6 hours, in the refrigerator for 6 days and in the freezer for 6 months. These numbers seem to be the easiest to remember. However, some sources will give different guidelines, such as 6-8 hours, 6-8 days and up to one year if you have a freezer temperature of 0 degrees Fahrenheit or colder. Use the guidelines you feel most comfortable with without wasting any milk. You worked hard to save that milk and your baby deserves every drop of it.

Expressed breast milk can be stored in glass, hard plastic or plastic freezer bags designed to store milk. Disposable bottle liners are not meant for storage as they often split or leak along the seams. The container should be labeled with the date and amount, unless it is pre-marked. Be sure to store milk in the back of the freezer where the temperature is coolest and most consistent. Consider storing in smaller portions of 2-4 ounces, to help decrease waste.

Breast milk is usually off-white or very light blue color. However the color can vary depending on what you've eaten or the time of day you pump. All shades of your milk are normal and should not affect the quality or taste of the milk. Like any fresh milk, your stored breast milk will separate with the fat rising to the top. Rotate or gently shake the container and the layers will mix evenly. This is not a sign your milk has gone bad.

Working and providing breast milk for your baby can be done successfully. It will take some planning, flexibility, commitment and a bit of patience. Give yourself some time to settle in to your new routine and always take a nap any chance you get. The sleepy relaxed feeling you have while you breastfeed can turn into a power nap for you. Learn to lie down to breastfeed, using the side-lying position.

In addition to caring for your baby, you now have a second job, as you return to your work responsibilities. You may find yourself feeling overwhelmed. This is a common feeling among new mothers, who for the most part find this feeling to be temporary. Be patient with yourself and your new routine. Each day will become easier. Hopefully your return to work and your baby starting to sleep longer each night will coincide. Surround yourself with people who will listen to you when you need support and will help you meet your breastfeeding goals.

Remember breastfeeding your baby is important and your commitment to it will be valued. Good luck and keep your dream alive to breastfeed as long as you and your baby desire.

My wish is you will find this book helpful as you navigate your way through your breastfeeding experience. It was written for you the mother, to help you along your journey. Take the time to enjoy this moment in your life. The moment of being a mom, breastfeeding your baby and creating a relationship like none you've ever known. It's an experience you will never forget. Congratulations and best of luck to you.

Bibliography

Books

Riordan, Jan; and Wambach, Karen; Breastfeeding and Human Lactation, 4th Edition , 2010. Jones and Bartlett, Publishing, Sundbury MA

Hale, Thomas W; Medications and Mothers' Milk, 15th Edition, 2012. Hale Publishing, Amarillo TX

Lawrence, Ruth; Breastfeeding: A guide for the Medical Profession 7th Edition, 2011 St Louis, MO; Mosby

AAP: Policy Statement; Breastfeeding and the Use of Human Milk, Pediatrics; Volume 129, Number 3, March 2012 Copyright © 2012 by the American Academy of Pediatrics

Walker, Marsha; Breastfeeding Management for the Clinician, 2nd Edition, 2011. Jones and Bartlett Publishing, Sundbury, MA

West, Diana; and Marasco, Lisa; The Breastfeeding Mother's Guide to Making More Milk, 2009 McGraw-Hill Companies

Marcu, Monica A (2005), Miracle Tree, KOS Health Publications, La Canada, CA.

Articles

Bergman, Dr Nils, Kangaroo Mother Care: Restoring the Original Paradigm for Infant Care and Breastfeeding, 2001

Collados-Gomez, L., Aragones-Corral, B., Contreras-Oliveras, I., Gracia-Feced, E., & Vila-Piqueras, M. (2011) Assessing the impact of kangaroo care on preterm infant stress. Enferecia Cinical, 21(2) 69-74.

Flacking, R., Ewald,U., & Wallin, U (2011) Positive effect of kangaroo mother care on long-term breastfeeding in very preterm infants. JOGNN, 40(2) 190-197.

Brandtzaeg P. The mucosal immune system and its integration with the mammary gland. The Journal of Pediatrics. 156(2,supplement 1) s8-s15. 2010By McGregor JA, Rogo LJ, Journal Of Human Lactation: Official Journal Of International Lactation Consultant Association [J Hum Lact], ISSN: 0890-3344, 2006 Aug; Vol. 22 (3), pp. 270-1; PMID: 16885486 Breast milk: an unappreciated source of stem cells.

By Shibata H, Yamane T, Aoyama Y, Nakamae H, Hasegawa T, Sakamoto C, Terada Y, Koh G, Hino M, Acta Haematologica [Acta Haematol], ISSN: 0001-5792, 2003; Vol. 110 (4), pp. 200-1; PMID: 14663166 Excretion of granulocyte colony-stimulating factor into human breast milk.

By Patki S, Kadam S, Chandra V, Bhonde R, Human Cell: Official Journal Of Human Cell Research Society [Hum Cell], ISSN: 1749-0774, 2010 May; Vol. 23 (2), pp. 35-40; PMID: 20712706 Human breast milk is a rich source of multipotent mesenchymal stem cells.

Websites

Academy of Breastfeeding Medicine
www.bfmed.org
American Academy of Family Health Care Providers
www.aapf.org
American Academy of Pediatrics
www.aap.org
Center for Lactation Education
www.bsccenter.org
International Lactation Consultant Association
www.ilca.org
La Leche League International
www.lalecheleague.org
Nursing Mothers Council
www.nursingmothers.org
World Health Organization
www.who.org
United States Breastfeeding Committee
www.usbreastfeeding.org

US Department of Health and Human Services
www.womenshealth.gov
Center for Disease Control
www.cdc.gov
Motherlove Herbal Company
www.motherlove.com
National Center for Biotechnology Information
www.ncbi.nih.gov
March of Dimes
www.marchofdimes.com
Brian Palmer, DDS
www.brianpalmerdds.com

Videos

Discovery Channel
www.youtube.com/channel/HC4QrBHUKx8R8
Jack Newman
www.youtube.com/watch?v=Wj9tLgYn-bA
Jack Newman
www.youtube.com/watch?v=VHs2QI5Kylo
stemcellworx.com.au
www.youtube.com/#/watch?v=KA6eO2fTEBQ
stemcellworx.com.au
www.youtube.com/watch?feature=relmfu&v=g_AHAwEE5s4

"When I first worked with Jill, I was amazed at the degree of passion, energy and enthusiasm she displayed in promoting that early bonding between the mother and her baby and establishing successful breast feeding. What impressed me most was her deep knowledge and calm approach in addressing any anxieties the parents may have to make it a truly exceptional experience!

Dr. Nancy Fahim, Neonatologist
University of Minnesota

Jill was wonderful to work with when I was learning to breastfeed my twins. She is friendly, easy to talk to and took the time to ask questions to learn our situation and then tailored her advice accordingly. I was not only impressed with the great solutions she provided for the issues I was struggling with but the amount of knowledge she had. She explained the whys behind her advice so I could better understand why the babies were doing what they were doing. I also appreciated that she was never pushy – she provided lots of options and let me decide what would work best for my family.

Haley Hemmen
New mother of twins Kylie and Cooper

About the Author

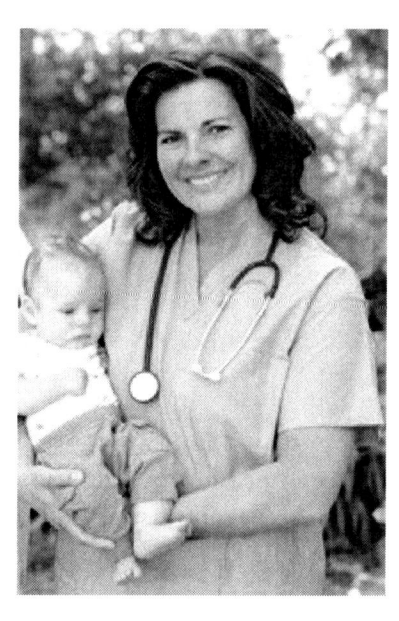

Jill Lindquist, RN.C, PHN, BSN, IBCLC

Her career has always centered around mothers and babies. With experience in antepartum, postpartum, nursery and home care case management, Jill understands what happens in and beyond the hospital. She has been board certified as a lactation consultant since 1995 and been a driving force for hospital based lactation programs and education. Her communication and teaching style has touched many families to help them have the breastfeeding experience they have always dreamed of having.